Atopic Dermatitis

Guest Editor

MARK BOGUNIEWICZ, MD

IMMUNOLOGY AND ALLERGY CLINICS OF NORTH AMERICA

www.immunology.theclinics.com

Consulting Editor
RAFEUL ALAM, MD, PhD

August 2010 • Volume 30 • Number 3

SAUNDERS an imprint of ELSEVIER, Inc.

W.B. SAUNDERS COMPANY
A Division of Elsevier Inc.

1600 John F. Kennedy Blvd., ● Suite 1800 ● Philadelphia, PA 19103-2899.

http://www.theclinics.com

IMMUNOLOGY AND ALLERGY CLINICS OF NORTH AMERICA Volume 30, Number 3
August 2010 ISSN 0889–8561, ISBN-13: 978-1-4377-2458-5

Editor: Patrick Manley

Immunology and Allergy Clinics of North America (ISSN 0889–8561) is published quarterly by Elsevier Inc., 360 Park Avenue South, New York, NY 10010-1710. Months of issue are February, May, August, and November. Periodicals postage paid at New York, NY and additional mailing offices. Subscription prices are $254.00 per year for US individuals, $373.00 per year for US institutions, $123.00 per year for US students and residents, $312.00 per year for Canadian individuals, $178.00 per year for Canadian students, $463.00 per year for Canadian institutions, $354.00 per year for international individuals, $463.00 per year for international institutions, $178.00 per year for international students. To receive student/resident rate, orders must be accompanied by name of affiliated institution, date of term, and the *signature* of program/residency coordinator on institution letterhead. Orders will be billed at individual rate until proof of status is received. Foreign air speed delivery is included in all *Clinics* subscription prices. All prices are subject to change without notice. **POSTMASTER**: Send address changes to *Immunology and Allergy Clinics of North America,* Elsevier Health Sciences Division, Subscription Customer Service, 3251 Riverport Lane, Maryland Heights, MO 63043. **Customer Service: 1-800-654-2452 (U.S. and Canada); 314-447-8871 (outside U.S. and Canada). Fax: 314-447-8029. E-mail: journalscustomerservice-usa@elsevier.com (for print support); journalsonlinesupport-usa@elsevier.com (for online support).**

Reprints. For copies of 100 or more, of articles in this publication, please contact the Commercial Reprints Department, Elsevier Inc., 360 Park Avenue South, New York, New York 10010-1710. Tel. (212) 633-3812, Fax: (212) 462-1935, e-mail: reprints@elsevier.com.

Immunology and Allergy Clinics of North America is covered in MEDLINE/PubMed (Index Medicus), Current Contents/Life Sciences, Science Citation Index, ISI/BIOMED, Chemical Abstracts, and EMBASE/Excerpta Medica.

Printed and bound by CPI Group (UK) Ltd, Croydon, CR0 4YY
Transferred to Digital Print 2011

Contributors

CONSULTING EDITOR

RAFEUL ALAM, MD, PhD
Veda and Chauncey Ritter Chair in Immunology, Professor, and Director, Division
of Immunology and Allergy, National Jewish Health; and University of Colorado
Health Sciences Center, Denver, Colorado

GUEST EDITOR

MARK BOGUNIEWICZ, MD
Professor, Division of Pediatric Allergy-Immunology, Department of Pediatrics,
National Jewish Health; and University of Colorado Denver School of Medicine,
Denver, Colorado

AUTHORS

MARCELLA R. AQUINO, MD
Clinical Instructor of Medicine, Department of Internal Medicine, State University
of New York at Stony Brook; Allergy and Immunology Attending, Division of
Rheumatology, Allergy and Immunology, Winthrop University Hospital, Mineola,
New York

BRUCE BENDER, PhD
Professor, Division of Pediatric Behavioral Health, National Jewish Health; Department
of Psychiatry, University of Colorado, Denver, Colorado

BRETT BIELORY, MD
Research Instructor, Department of Ophthalmology, Bascom Palmer Eye Institute,
University of Miami Miller School of Medicine, Miami, Florida

LEONARD BIELORY, MD
Director, Medicine, Pediatrics and Ophthalmology, STARx Allergy and Asthma Center,
Springfield; Professor, Center for Climate Prediction, Rutgers University, New Brunswick,
New Jersey

MARK BOGUNIEWICZ, MD
Professor, Division of Pediatric Allergy-Immunology, Department of Pediatrics,
National Jewish Health; and University of Colorado Denver School of Medicine,
Denver, Colorado

JEAN-CHRISTOPH CAUBET, MD
University Hospitals of Geneva; University of Geneva Medical School, Geneva,
Switzerland; Fellow, Division of Pediatric Allergy and Immunology, Mount Sinai
School of Medicine, New York, New York

SARAH L. CHAMLIN, MD
Associate Professor of Pediatrics and Dermatology, Division of Pediatric Dermatology, Children's Memorial Hospital; Department of Dermatology, Northwestern's Feinberg School of Medicine, Chicago, Illinois

MARY-MARGARET CHREN, MD
Professor, Department of Dermatology, University of California at San Francisco, San Francisco, California

PHILIPPE A. EIGENMANN, MD
University Hospitals of Geneva; University of Geneva Medical School, Geneva, Switzerland

STEVEN J. ERSSER, PhD (Lond), RN, CertTHEd
Professor of Nursing Development and Skin Care Research; Director, Centre for Wellbeing and Quality of Life, School of Health and Social Care, Bournemouth University, Bournemouth; Member, Nursing Advisory Board, International Skin Care Nursing Group, London, United Kingdom

LUZ S. FONACIER, MD
Professor of Clinical Medicine, Department of Internal Medicine, State University of New York at Stony Brook; Program Director, Allergy and Immunology Fellowship; Section Head of Allergy, Division of Rheumatology, Allergy and Immunology, Winthrop University Hospital, Mineola, New York

KIMBERLY KELSAY, MD
Associate Professor, Division of Pediatric Behavioral Health, National Jewish Health; Department of Psychiatry, University of Colorado, Denver, Colorado

MARY KLINNERT, PhD
Associate Professor, Division of Pediatric Behavioral Health, National Jewish Health; Department of Psychiatry, University of Colorado, Denver, Colorado

JOOHEE LEE, MD
Resident Physician, Department of Internal Medicine, Mayo Clinic, Rochester, Minnesota

DONALD Y.M. LEUNG, MD, PhD
Edelstein Chair of Pediatric Allergy and Immunology, National Jewish Health; Professor, Department of Pediatrics, University of Colorado Denver, Denver, Colorado

NOREEN HEER NICOL, MS, RN, FNP
Director, Professional Development, The Children's Hospital; PhD Candidate, University of Colorado - Clinical Sciences; Senior Clinical Instructor, University of Colorado, Denver, Colorado; Member, Nursing Advisory Board, International Skin Care Nursing Group, London, United Kingdom

PECK Y. ONG, MD
Assistant Professor of Clinical Pediatrics, Division of Clinical Immunology and Allergy, Childrens Hospital Los Angeles; Department of Pediatrics, Keck School of Medicine, University of Southern California, Los Angeles, California

CHRISTINA SCHNOPP, MD
Department of Dermatology and Allergy, Technical University, Munich, Germany

DANIEL A. SEARING, MD
Fellow, Division of Pediatric Allergy and Immunology, Department of Pediatrics,
National Jewish Health, Denver, Colorado

JONATHAN M. SPERGEL, MD, PhD
Associate Professor of Pediatrics; Chief, Allergy Section, Division of Allergy and
Immunology, The Children's Hospital of Philadelphia, University of Pennsylvania
School of Medicine, Philadelphia, Pennsylvania

ANDREAS WOLLENBERG, MD, FAAAAI
Department of Dermatology and Allergy, Ludwig-Maximilian University, Munich,
Germany

Contents

Atopic dermatitis (AD) is one of the most common chronic childhood skin diseases affecting up to 17% of children in the United States. The point prevalence of AD has increased based on validated questionnaires in the most recent update of the International Study of Asthma and Allergies in Childhood. However, the increases are primarily in developing countries, whereas the rates have stabilized in countries with higher incomes. AD starts in early childhood with 65% of children affected by 18 months of age. Furthermore, less than half of the patients with AD have complete resolution by 7 years of age and only 60% have resolution by adulthood, indicating the chronic nature of AD. AD is a major risk factor for the development of asthma, with an increased odds ratio in children with AD in several longitudinal studies compared with children without AD, and about 30% of patients with AD develop asthma. Patients with atopic sensitization along with eczema are at a higher risk for progressing in the atopic march to asthma. The main risk factors for progression and persistence of asthma are early onset and severity of AD.

Atopic dermatitis is a common childhood skin disease of increasing prevalence that greatly affects the quality-of-life of affected children and their families. The complex and multidimensional effects of this disease have been described qualitatively and measured quantitatively with quality-of-life instruments. The burden of atopic dermatitis can likely be improved by identifying parents and their caregivers with impaired quality-of-life and providing appropriate education and psychosocial support.

Food or environmental allergens play a significant pathogenic role in a subgroup of patients with atopic dermatitis (AD) and can trigger eczema flares. This review focuses on when and which diagnostic and allergen-avoidance measures are beneficial. Diagnosis of allergic triggers may be aided by skin-prick tests measuring serum-specific IgE and/or atopy patch tests (APT) based on the patient's history, and when necessary, oral food challenges (OFC). In a subset of patients, therapeutic measures, such as elimination of the incriminated allergen(s), can lead to marked improvement of AD; this is especially true for food allergens, but can also apply to inhalant allergens.

Atopic dermatitis is characterized by *Staphylococcus aureus* colonization and recurrent skin infections. In addition to an increased risk of invasive infections by herpes simplex or vaccinia viruses, there is ample evidence that microbial pathogens, particularly *S aureus* and fungi, contribute to the cutaneous inflammation of atopic dermatitis. The authors describe recent developments in the pathogenesis of atopic dermatitis in relation to the role of microbial pathogens. Understanding how microbial pathogens interact or evade the cutaneous immunity of atopic dermatitis may be crucial in preventing infections or cutaneous inflammation in this disease.

Atopic dermatitis, a chronic disease seen by allergist-immunologists, has both dermatologic and ocular manifestations. The ocular component is often disproportionately higher than the dermatologic disease. Even if skin abnormalities seem well controlled, these patients require ophthalmic evaluation. Atopic keratoconjunctivitis in atopic dermatitis patients is characterized by acute exacerbations and requires maintenance therapy for long-term control. Future studies will continue to emphasize the use of steroid-sparing, immunomodulating agents that have the potential to provide long-lasting anti-inflammatory control with a more favorable side-effect profile.

Although allergic contact dermatitis (CD) was previously thought to occur less frequently in patients with atopic dermatitis (AD), more recent studies show that it is at least as common in patients with AD as in the general population, if not more so. Thus, patients with AD should be considered for patch testing (PT). Although conflicting data exist, the severity of the AD may impact the PT results. Furthermore, younger patients may yield more positive PT results. Hand eczema and compositae allergy are more common in atopic patients. Reassuringly, PT is positive for topical antiseptic and corticosteroids in only a small subset of patients. When personal products are patch tested, emollients should be included in the series.

Conventional therapy for atopic dermatitis has evolved along with better understanding of underlying impaired barrier function, role of microorganisms, and immune abnormalities. Emollients, along with antimicrobial and topical anti-inflammatory therapies, remain the cornerstone of conventional therapy. Recent therapeutic advances include use of nonsteroidal therapy for epidermal barrier repair, along with proactive therapy with topical corticosteroids and calcineurin inhibitors. Minimal anti-inflammatory treatment of the underlying residual disease is the immunobiologic rationale for proactive therapy. Further progress in understanding this increasingly common disease will hopefully lead to more targeted therapies.

Nursing is making a key contribution to the development and evaluation of atopic dermatitis (AD) education. Educational interventions have long been recommended and used as a critical adjunct at all levels of therapy for patients with AD to enhance therapy effectiveness. These interventions may be directed toward adult patients or the parent/caregiver or child with eczema. Education should be individualized and includes teaching about the chronic or relapsing nature of AD, exacerbating factors, and therapeutic options with benefits, risks, and realistic expectations. This important educational facet of care management is becoming increasingly difficult to accomplish in routine care visits and seems to be equally difficult to measure and evaluate. A limited number of studies to date suggest effectiveness of educational approaches to improve the management of AD. We recommend that an international priority be given to assessing the effects of patient and parental education by nurses and other care providers in AD management using research studies designed to address the common weaknesses of existing randomized studies and the relative benefits of different strategies.

Moderate to severe atopic dermatitis (AD) negatively affects patients and their families. Pruritus, scratching, and sleep problems are common complaints linked to disturbed quality of life. Treatment is complex, and nonadherence rates are high. This article reviews the effect of AD on patients and their families and intervention strategies that have some success in improving quality of life. A treatment model for addressing the psychosocial effect of moderate to severe AD within a multidisciplinary setting is suggested herein.

This review examines the scientific evidence behind the hypothesis that vitamin D plays a role in the pathogenesis of allergic diseases, along with a focus on emerging data regarding vitamin D and atopic dermatitis. Elucidated molecular interactions of vitamin D with components of the immune system and clinical data regarding vitamin D deficiency and atopic diseases are discussed. The rationale behind the sunshine hypothesis, laboratory evidence supporting links between vitamin D deficiency and allergic diseases, the clinical evidence for and against vitamin D playing a role in allergic diseases, and the emerging evidence regarding the potential use of vitamin D to augment the innate immune response in atopic dermatitis are reviewed.

The burden of atopic diseases, including atopic dermatitis (AD), is significant and far-reaching. In addition to cost of care and therapies, it affects the quality of life for those affected as well as their caretakers. Complementary and alternative therapies are commonly used because of concerns about potential adverse effects of conventional therapies and frustration with the lack of response to prescribed medications, be it due to the severity of the AD or the lack of appropriate regular use. Despite the promising results reported with various herbal medicines and biologic products, the clinical efficacy of such alternative therapies remains to be determined. Physicians need to be educated about alternative therapies and discuss benefits and potential adverse effects or limitations with patients. A systematic approach and awareness of reputable and easily accessible resources are helpful in dealing with complementary and alternative medicine (CAM). The use of CAM interventions is common among individuals with AD. Epidemiologic data have been a motivating drive for better elucidation of the efficacy of CAM interventions for allergic disease. Herbal medicines and biologics for AD treatment and, more recently, prevention comprise a major area of clinical investigation. Potential mechanisms of therapeutic effect elucidated by animal models and human clinical studies implicate modulation of TH2-type allergic inflammation and induction of immune tolerance. Population-based research regarding the use of CAM for allergic diseases underscores the increasing challenge for care providers with respect to identifying CAM use and ensuring safe use of allopathic and complementary medicines in disease management.

Atopic dermatitis can be a challenging disease to treat, often having a chronic or relapsing course. For patients with moderate to severe disease, it can result in significant morbidity and affect quality of life of patients or families. Current treatment can be associated with side effects or patient and caregiver concerns about use. Recent advances in the understanding of barrier defects and innate and adaptive immune systemic abnormalities in atopic dermatitis have provided potential new targets for therapeutic intervention. These advances include antimicrobial peptides, antistaphylococcal toxin strategies, Th2 cytokine inhibitors, and modulation of pruritus at the neuromediator level.

RELATED INTEREST

Pediatric Clinics of North America (Volume 57, Issue 1, Pages 1–352, February 2010)
Hematopoietic Stem Cell Transplantation
Max J. Coppes, MD, PhD, MBA, Terry J. Fry, MD, and Crystal L. Mackall, MD,
Guest Editors

THE CLINICS ARE NOW AVAILABLE ONLINE!

Access your subscription at:
www.theclinics.com

Foreword
Atopic Dermatitis

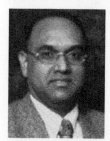

Rafeul Alam, MD, PhD
Consulting Editor

The difference between atopic dermatitis and other atopic illnesses is that the pathologic process in the former can be followed visually from the start to the end. Unlike other organs affected by atopic conditions, skin can be inspected on an ongoing basis, biopsied at various stages, and intervened pharmacologically more easily. This makes atopic dermatitis an excellent model disease to study. Because of this easy accessibility, atopic dermatitis has provided exciting new knowledge to the field of allergy over the years. It is a disease where Th1, Th2, and Th17 cells work in an orderly sequence to produce a complete phenotype. The high prevalence of filagrin mutation in atopic dermatitis suggests that structural abnormalities leading to tissue permeability play an important role in the clinical manifestation of the disease.[1] Tissue permeability altering the threshold for inflammation seems to be a unifying theme not only for atopic dermatitis and asthma but also for chronic enterocolitis. The identification of thymic stromal lymphopoietin (TSLP) as a permeability-promoting cytokine[2] and IL-31 as a pruritogenic cytokine[3] is likely to have therapeutic implications. Thanks to the advances in genomic studies, we have a better understanding of the mechanism of chronic bacterial colonization of the skin in atopic dermatitis.[4] Some of the observations made in atopic dermatitis are likely to have relevance for diseases such as asthma.

Drs Donald Leung and Mark Boguniewicz have been pioneering basic investigations in atopic dermatitis for many years. Under the editorial guidance of

---

This work was supported by NIH Grants RO1 AI059719 and AI68088, PPG HL 36577, and N01 HHSN272200700048C.

Immunol Allergy Clin N Am 30 (2010) xiii–xiv
doi:10.1016/j.iac.2010.06.009
0889-8561/10/$ – see front matter

immunology.theclinics.com

Dr Boguniewicz, this issue presents the state-of-the-art of basic and clinical science in atopic dermatitis.

Rafeul Alam, MD, PhD
Division of Allergy & Immunology
National Jewish Health & University of Colorado
Denver Health Sciences Center
1400 Jackson Street, Denver, CO 80206, USA

E-mail address:
alamr@njc.org

REFERENCES

1. Palmer CN, Irvine AD, Terron-Kwiatkowski A, et al. Common loss-of-function variants of the epidermal barrier protein filaggrin are a major predisposing factor for atopic dermatitis. Nat Genet 2006;38:441–6.
2. Liu YJ. Thymic stromal lymphopoietin: master switch for allergic inflammation. J Exp Med 2006;203:269–73.
3. Dillon SR, Sprecher C, Hammond A, et al. Interleukin 31, a cytokine produced by activated T cells, induces dermatitis in mice. Nat Immunol 2004;5(7):752–60.
4. Ong PY, Ohtake T, Brandt C, et al. Endogenous antimicrobial peptides and skin infections in atopic dermatitis. N Engl J Med 2002;347:1151–60.

Preface
Atopic Dermatitis

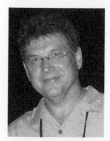

Mark Boguniewicz, MD
Guest Editor

Since the last issue of *Immunology and Allergy Clinics of North America* devoted to atopic dermatitis was published in 2002, a number of important observations have been made regarding our understanding of the underlying pathophysiology of this disease and new approaches, including a change in the treatment paradigm, have emerged based on these insights. I am pleased that the Consulting Editor, Dr Rafeul Alam, has identified atopic dermatitis as an important disease worthy of a timely review devoted to these advances and I am honored to once again serve as Editor for the Atopic Dermatitis issue. I wish to express my sincere gratitude to the distinguished group of authors who generously agreed to share their expertise and valuable time in contributing to these state-of-the-art reviews. These internationally recognized experts address a diverse range of relevant topics including epidemiology, triggers and confounding problems, basic and clinical research, therapeutic approaches, as well as education of patients and caregivers. Atopic dermatitis remains an all too common disease with a global presence that significantly impacts the quality of life of patients and their families and places a heavy financial burden on our society. Importantly, it frequently precedes the development of allergies and asthma, and a growing appreciation of the complex relationship between epidermal barrier and immune abnormalities provides a rationale for early identification of the subset of patients whose phenotype includes early-onset, severe, and persistent atopic dermatitis associated with allergic sensitization and recurrent wheezing as well as a proactive approach to therapy. This issue should prove valuable to readers with interest in basic mechanisms of atopic dermatitis as well as clinical care of patients with this disease.

Mark Boguniewicz, MD
Division of Pediatric Allergy-Immunology, Department of Pediatrics
National Jewish Health and University of Colorado School of Medicine
1400 Jackson Street, J310
Denver, CO 80206, USA

E-mail address:
boguniewiczm@njhealth.org

Immunol Allergy Clin N Am 30 (2010) xv
doi:10.1016/j.iac.2010.06.008   immunology.theclinics.com
0889-8561/10/$ – see front matter © 2010 Elsevier Inc. All rights reserved.

Epidemiology of Atopic Dermatitis and Atopic March in Children

Jonathan M. Spergel, MD, PhD

KEYWORDS

- Atopic dermatitis • Atopic march • Epidemiology

Epidemiology (derived from the Greek terms *epi* meaning upon, among; *demos* meaning people, district; and *logos* meaning study, word, discourse) is the study of what is upon people.[1] In medicine, it refers to diseases that are affecting people and the study of factors affecting an illness. There are several ways to examine the epidemiology of a disease. Studies can include the prevalence (total number of active cases) or the incidence (risk of new cases) of a disease. By examining these 2 factors, the natural history of a disease can be studied. This review focuses on the prevalence and natural history of atopic dermatitis (AD).

PREVALENCE OF AD

Prevalence has been examined in different ways with each having its own benefits and faults. The most accurate way is an expert physician diagnosis of all patients in a community. However, this is labor intensive and not practical on a larger scale. Another approach is to pick a random population and have an expert physician confirm the diagnosis and estimate population prevalence based on a small subset of patients. This approach has the inherent problem of scaling the conclusion based on a small population. A third approach is to use the *International Classification of Diseases, Ninth Revision* (ICD-9) codes to estimate the prevalence based on medical records. However, ICD-9 codes are neither universally used nor always coded correctly. The fourth approach is to base prevalence on standardized questionnaires given to physicians or families to determine diagnosis. The questionnaires are validated based on physician history and physical examination. This method has been used for most worldwide prevalence data.[2,3] The International Study of Asthma and Allergies in Childhood (ISAAC) is a worldwide epidemiologic research program established in 1991 using this technique. It has been used in 3 different phases and in more

Division of Allergy and Immunology, The Children's Hospital of Philadelphia, University of Pennsylvania School of Medicine, 3550 Market Street, Philadelphia, PA 19104, USA
E-mail address: spergel@email.chop.edu

Immunol Allergy Clin N Am 30 (2010) 269–280
doi:10.1016/j.iac.2010.06.003
0889-8561/10/$ – see front matter © 2010 Elsevier Inc. All rights reserved.

than 100 countries. The most recent completed phase was done in 245 collaborating centers in 99 countries with a total of 1,187,496 children participating. The prevalence was determined in 2 age groups (6–7 and 13–14 years). In the 13- to 14-year age group, 233 centers from 97 countries participated, and in the 6- to 7-year age group, there were 144 collaborating centers participating from 61 countries. For AD or flexural eczema, 3 questions were asked to the families in their native language. Children were classified as having had flexural eczema in the past 12 months if their parents answered yes to 2 of the 3 following questions: "Has your child ever had an itchy rash which was coming and going for at least 6 months?" "Has your child had this itchy rash at any time in the last 12 months?" and "Has this itchy rash at any time affected any of the following places: folds of the elbows, behind the knees, in front of the ankles, under the buttocks, or around the neck, ears, or eyes?"[4] A high correlation between answering yes to 2 questions and the diagnosis of flexural eczema has been found.[2,5,6]

Studies by ISAAC have found 60-fold variation in prevalence of flexural eczema, ranging from 0.3% to 20.5%.[2,5] Examination of prevalence across the world reveals some interesting findings (**Fig. 1**).[2,3] The prevalence of eczema is higher in wealthy nations, and there are pockets of high prevalence in countries with lower incomes, suggesting multiple causes for the existence of eczema.

The ISAAC study also found an increase in AD in both the age groups (6–7 and 13–14 years) albeit in only a 7-year period because phase III was a repeat of phase I.[6] There was a significant increase in the prevalence of AD, ranging from 0.07% to 1.09% in 48 countries with decrease in 8 countries and little change in 12 countries in the 6- to 7-year age group and increase in 47 countries, decrease in 32 countries, and little change in 26 countries in the 13- to 14-year age group (**Fig. 2**). Overall, the increase in prevalence occurred primarily in previous areas of low prevalence, whereas the areas with previous high levels showed leveling off.[6,7] These results raise the question whether the increase is caused by increased recognition or other changes in

Atopic Dermatitis

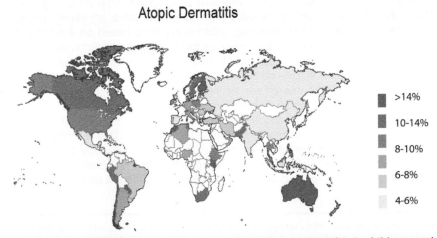

>14%

10-14%

8-10%

6-8%

4-6%

Fig. 1. Prevalence of AD in the world based on ISAAC Phase 1–3 studies in children aged 13 to 14 years. (*Data* from Asher MI, Montefort S, Bjorksten B, et al. Worldwide time trends in the prevalence of symptoms of asthma, allergic rhinoconjunctivitis, and eczema in childhood: ISAAC Phases One and Three repeat multicountry cross-sectional surveys. Lancet 2006;368:733–43.)

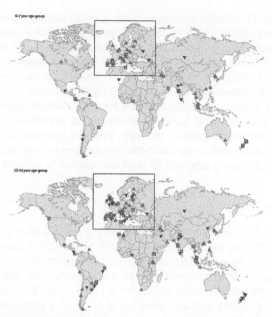

Fig. 2. World map showing direction of change in the prevalence of eczema for 6- to 7-year and 13- to 14-year age groups. Each symbol represents a center. ∇, prevalence reduced by 1 SE per year; $\square$, little change; $\triangle$, prevalence increased by 1 SE per year. (*From* Asher MI, Montefort S, Bjorksten B, et al. Worldwide time trends in the prevalence of symptoms of asthma, allergic rhinoconjunctivitis, and eczema in childhood: ISAAC Phases One and Three repeat multicountry cross-sectional surveys. Lancet 2006;368:740; with permission.)

environment, because the period of 7 years is too short for major genetic or ecological changes.

In a population-based study from the United States, the prevalence of eczema among children aged 5 to 9 years was estimated at 17.2% in Oregon schoolchildren, which is consistent with ISAAC data.[8] Estimates were based on questionnaires that were validated by physical examination of select children. Based on strict criteria of a physician diagnosis, the prevalence was found to be 6.8%. A similar nationwide survey was done in 60,000 households in the United States. The survey had a 70% response rate representing 116,000 individuals, with eczema in 1 of the 4 areas in the body in 17% of the individuals and defined eczema in 10.7%.[9] These results are similar to that of the studies by ISAAC, indicating the prevalence to be between 10% and 20% in the United States depending on the diagnostic criteria.

IS AD ATOPIC?

There is a debate whether AD is truly linked to atopy. The most recent ISAAC study suggests a possible answer for differences observed in previous results. Studies have shown either no link or a link or possible link between atopy and atopic AD.

In the ISAAC phase II study, 32,205 schoolchildren aged 8 to 12 years from 20 countries were examined for flexural eczema and also had skin prick testing done to both species of dust mite (*Dermatophagoides pteronyssinus, Dermatophagoides farinae*), cat hair, *Alternaria tenuis*, mixed tree and grass pollens, and allergens of local relevance.[4] Among 17 affluent countries (with a gross national per capital income >$9200), 13 had statistically significant odds ratios (ORs) for a positive association between flexural eczema and atopy with a combined OR of 2.69. In the nonaffluent countries, only 2 of 13 countries (Estonia and India) had a borderline positive association, and combined countries had an OR of 1.17. The OR for the association of atopy with flexural eczema plotted against income was highly significant ($P = .006$). Another way to answer this question is to observe the fraction of atopic patients with flexural eczema, which was 27.9% and 1.2% for affluent- and nonaffluent-country centers, respectively. This fraction suggests multiple types of flexural eczema (an allergic type in affluent countries and nonatopic type in nonaffluent countries) that are consistent with the data of finding pockets of high prevalence in affluent and nonaffluent countries.

NATURAL HISTORY OF AD

An important aspect of the natural history of AD is the number and percentage of patients who will outgrow their disease. Ricci and colleagues[10] studied 205 children, who were followed up from 6 to 36 months to 22 to 27 years of age by a standardized questionnaire. Overall, 60% reported that their eczema resolved, with the patients with severe AD reporting a longer time to resolution (6 years of age for severe and 5.5 years of age for mild AD). Patients with egg allergy and AD tended to take longer to outgrow their AD.

The Multicenter Allergy Study (MAS) followed up a birth cohort of 1314 children in Germany.[11] The study classified the outcome in 3 age categories into 3 groups (intermittent, resolution, and persistent). It was found that 13.4% of the studied population had AD by 1 year of age and 21.5% of patients had AD by 2 years of age. At 7 years of age, 43% were in complete remission, 38% had an intermittent pattern, and 19% had persistent symptoms, with more than half of the patients with AD showing some signs of the disease past 7 years of age. Risk factors for persistent AD were initial severity (OR 5.86) and atopic sensitization (OR 2.76), with severity being the strongest risk factor identified.[11]

In the ALSPAC (Avon Longitudinal Study of Parents and Children) study, 1509 randomly selected children were followed up from birth to 5 years of age.[12] Among them, 495 (33%) had early-onset AD before 18 months of age, 273 (18%) had onset after 18 months of age, and 429 (49%) were not affected. Only 2% had eczema at every study visit (1, 6, 18, 30, and 42 months). The study classified 40% of children as intermittent (symptoms of some of the clinical visits) early-onset AD and 22% as intermittent late-onset AD, with 35% affected at 4 years of age. The risk factor identified in this study for persistent AD was elevated serum IgE levels at 12 months of age. Similar to the MAS, there was a higher rate of AD in this population than reported in the ISAAC study, suggesting a higher rate if physician diagnosis is used rather than questionnaires. Also, the rate of resolution was similar, indicating that 30% to 40% of children still had AD in early school-age years.

ATOPIC MARCH

Patients with AD may develop a typical sequence of food allergy, rhinitis, and asthma, which develop at certain ages; some may persist for several years, whereas others may resolve with increasing age.[13] This progression of atopic manifestations from AD to allergic rhinitis to asthma is known as the atopic march (**Fig. 3**), which has been supported by several cross-sectional and longitudinal studies (**Table 1**).[10,14,15,17–22,24] In a review, van der Hulst and colleagues[21] examined

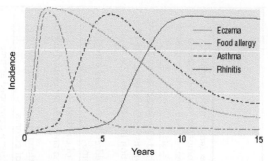

Fig. 3. Progression of the atopic march. (*From* Barnetson RS, Rogers M. Childhood atopic eczema. BMJ 2002;324:1376; with permission.)

13 cohort studies, 4 birth studies, and 9 cohort studies on children with eczema from 1950 to 2006 for this link. The investigators found an OR of 2.14 for developing asthma after eczema compared with children without eczema. In this analysis, approximately 30% of children with eczema developed asthma.

In a close examination at some of the pivotal trials, the Tucson Children's Respiratory Study found that 18% of children with wheezing at 6 years of age had eczema before 2 years of age.[14] The cohort has now reached 22 years of age, and childhood asthma is associated with eczema, whereas adult-onset asthma is not.[23] Also, the increased risk of developing asthma in a patient with eczema may be true only for the subgroup with specific IgE to aeroallergens, because 2 studies found a significantly stronger association with asthma for atopic eczema compared with nonatopic eczema.[18,20] This large study also supports a particular phenotype of allergic eczema that progresses into an allergic phenotype of asthma.

In addition, the Tucson Children's Respiratory Study has developed an asthma predictive index, which includes physician-diagnosed AD and allergic sensitization as part of the criteria for risk factors of asthma.[24] The asthma predictive index has a modest positive predictive value of 47.5% at 6 years of age and an excellent negative predicative value of 91.6%. Further evidence for the linkage of atopy, AD, and asthma showed that children with atopy have decreased lung function at 3 years of age.[25]

The MAS also found a relationship between atopy, eczema, and wheezing similar to the previous 2 studies.[15] Illi and colleagues[16] suggested that eczema and early wheezing were a separate phenotype and not part of the atopic march. The investigators found that early eczema without early wheezing was not associated with increased wheezing at 7 years of age. However, the risk for developing asthma was higher in children with early eczema and atopic sensitization (OR 6.68) than the association of early eczema with wheezing (OR 2.84).[26] These studies suggest that atopy along with eczema is a major risk factor for progression in the atopic march as shown in the Tucson Study.

In addition, severity of eczema is another risk factor because Gustafsson and colleagues[17] found that more than 50% of young children with severe AD ultimately developed asthma and approximately 75% developed allergic rhinitis. Similarly, Ricci and colleagues[10] followed up 252 children with AD and found that 33% of those with mild AD developed asthma when compared with 25% with moderate AD and 59% with severe AD. The OR for developing asthma adjusted to mild being 1 was 2.59 for moderate AD and 4.77 for severe AD.

Table 1
Studies examining eczema and development of asthma

Study	Patient Population	Major Findings
Martinez et al, 1995[14]	Birth cohort of 826 children in Tucson, Arizona, upto 6 y of age	• OR 2.4 risk factor for eczema for developing persistent wheezing compared with noneczema • 18% of persistent wheezers had asthma compared with 7.7% of nonwheezers
Kulig et al, 1999[15] and Illi et al, 2001[16]	1314 newborn infants in 5 German cities; followed up at 7 y	• By age 5 y, 69% who had developed AD by 3 mo of age were sensitized against aeroallergens; rate of aeroallergen sensitization increased to 77% in all high-risk children • By age 5 y, 50% of children with AD had allergic airway disease or asthma
Gustafsson et al, 2000[17]	94 children with AD, aged 4–35 mo at recruitment, followed up to age 7 y	• AD resolved in 35.1% of children • 43% developed asthma and 45% developed allergic rhinitis • Risk of developing asthma was higher in children with a family history of eczema
Novembre et al, 2001[18]	77 children with AD, aged 2–11 y	• 59% of early atopy/eczema developed asthma compared with 25% of late atopy/eczema and 0% of nonatopic eczema
Ohshima et al, 2002[19]	169 Japanese infants with AD followed up for 4 y	• 35% had developed asthma by the end of the study
Wuthrich and Schmid-Grendelmeier, 2002[20]	22 children with AD, 2–4 y to 10–12 y	• 60% of the children with atopic eczema developed asthma compared with 14% of children with nonatopic eczema

Ricci et al, 2006[10]	252 children with AD, aged 6–36 mo, followed up until remission or stabilization of AD	• AD disappeared in 60.5% of cases • Average age for recovery was 6 y for severe, 5.8 y for moderate, and 5.5 y for mild form of AD • Asthma developed in 34.1% of cases and rhinoconjunctivitis in 57.6% • Severity of AD is predicable for the onset of asthma
Porsbjerg et al, 2006[48]	291-patient cohort, followed up from 7–17 y to 19–29 y of age	• Eczema predicted the development of asthma (OR 3.2)
van der Hulst et al, 2007[21]	3103 patients from 4 birth cohort studies and 2278 patients from 9 eczema cohort studies	• Risk of developing asthma was elevated in young children with AD in the birth cohort studies (OR 2.14; 95% CI, 1.67–2.75) • Prevalence of asthma at age 6 y in eczema cohort studies was 35.8% among inpatients and 29.5% in a group of both inpatients and outpatients • About 1 of 3 children with eczema experienced asthma in later childhood
Kapoor et al, 2008[22]	2270 children with physician-confirmed AD, aged 2–17 y, living in the United States	• 33.3% had symptoms of only asthma or allergic rhinitis • 38% had symptoms of asthma and allergic rhinitis • Nearly 66% of children reported an additional form of AD by age 3 y (ie, atopic triad)
Stern et al, 2008[23]	849 birth cohort, followed up to 22 y of age	• Eczema by 2 y of age had OR of 3.8 for chronic asthma compared with 2.0 for inactive asthma

Abbreviation: CI, confidence interval.

MODELS FOR ATOPIC MARCH

Environmental and genetic evidence suggest that a defect in epithelial barrier integrity may contribute to the onset of AD and progression of the atopic march.[27] The integrity of the barrier, which controls the transcutaneous movement of water and prevents entry of external irritants, microbes, and allergens, is assessed by measuring transepidermal water loss. Impairment of the epithelial barrier function has been shown via an increase in transepidermal water loss in both lesioned skin and clinically unaffected skin in AD.[28] Epidermal skin barrier's integrity and function may be impaired by a range of irritants and allergens, which may lead to cytokine production, inflammation, and the development of eczematous lesions.

The likelihood that epidermal barrier dysfunction can initiate systemic sensitization and increase the risk of asthma and other allergic diseases is supported by experimental data, with the progression from allergic rhinitis to asthma or from AD to asthma in mouse models.[29–31] In these murine models, T cells have been shown to be critical because sensitization does not occur in the absence of $T\alpha\beta$ cells but does occur without B cells, IL-4, IL-5, and interferon gamma.[32–34] In addition, a key role for thymic stromal lymphopoietin (TSLP) has been hypothesized. TSLP is highly expressed in the skin of sensitized mice, and its deletion prevents the atopic march from occurring.[35] Furthermore, the importance of expression of TSLP in the skin is underscored because the expression of TSLP in the peripheral blood does not lead to development of the asthma phenotype, while the induction of TSLP with topical application of a vitamin D analogue leads to a murine model of the atopic march and asthma.[36] IL-17 also has an important role in these murine models, because it is necessary for the induction of airway hyperresponsiveness.[37]

GENETIC SUPPORT FOR ATOPIC MARCH

Epithelial barrier defects derived from loss-of-function mutations in the filaggrin gene have been identified as a strong predisposing factor for AD as well as for other inflammatory conditions, such as ichthyosis vulgaris.[38,39] The filaggrin gene encodes profilaggrin, a highly phosphorylated protein found in the keratohyalin granules in the granular layer of the outer epidermis. Mutations of the filaggrin genes can lead to impaired keratinization and defects in the epidermal barrier and thus probable increase to allergen sensitization.[40,41]

Smith and colleagues[41] were the first to show that loss-of-function mutations, R501X and 2282del4, in the filaggrin gene were responsible for ichthyosis vulgaris in 15 families, which is the most common inherited disorder of keratinization. Based on the results, it was estimated that these mutations were present in 9% of the European population.[38] Subsequent studies and a comprehensive meta-analysis have confirmed both the filaggrin polymorphisms as major risk factors for AD.[42–45] Although research shows a significant association of the 2 filaggrin mutations with asthma and allergic rhinitis, there is no apparent association between filaggrin and asthma without the coexistence of AD.[38] In a subgroup of German children participating in the ISAAC study, filaggrin variants increased the risk more than 3-fold for AD and more than 2-fold for allergic rhinitis independent of AD.[44] Of course, ascertaining the precise contribution of filaggrin mutations to the overall prevalence of these atopic diseases is confounded by temporal and disease severity factors in conjunction with putative environmental effects. The theory is that filaggrin leads to a leaky skin layer allowing penetration of allergen leading to sensitization. This sensitization is seen as positive skin test (atopy), and leaky skin barrier leads to AD. The subsequent sensitization through T cells and TSLP leads to development of asthma. This model is supported by circumstantial evidence (association of AD and atopy and the development of asthma) in the MAS, Ricci and colleagues',[10] and Tucson studies.[11,46] Also, the genetic evidence of the association between filaggrin, asthma, and atopy is supported by this model.[47]

SUMMARY

AD is one of the most common pediatric skin disorders with a prevalence of 20% in several studies.[8] The actual incidence is hard to estimate because most studies have examined point prevalence. AD like many other atopic diseases has increased in occurrence in the last couple of decades. However, the increase seems to be stabilizing in developed countries, with most of the current increase in areas with low prevalence in the past.[6] There is a difference in the relationship between atopy and eczema in countries with higher and lower incomes. The wealthier countries show a strong relationship between flexural eczema and atopy, which was not seen in the poorer countries based on family income and skin testing.[7] This finding along with differences in prevalence suggests different flexural eczema or AD phenotypes.

The natural history of AD has also been clarified over the last several years. Although previously AD was thought to resolve, recent longitudinal studies indicate that about 50% of patients with AD have intermittent symptoms until 7 years of age. Also, most patients with AD have symptoms early in life (<24 months of age). The natural history of AD is also associated with the development of other atopic diseases. Almost every study that examined this feature has found similar salient points. About 30% of the patients may develop asthma, whereas nearly 66% develop allergic sensitization and symptoms of allergic rhinitis.[11] The studies have also consistently found about a 2-fold increase in OR for development of asthma, which increases with AD severity.[17]

The discovery of the filaggrin gene and the relationships between filaggrin mutations and AD and murine models and the development of asthma from AD have suggested a potential model of pathogenesis. A proposed model is that the filaggrin mutations in susceptible patients (or other variation in the epidermal differentiation layer of the skin) lead to increased barrier disruption,[41] transepidermal water loss, and increased penetration of allergens and/or microorganisms (due to decreased synthesis of antimicrobial peptides).[48] These allergens along with microorganisms cause a T_H2 sensitization that is dependent on TSLP.[32,33,35] The T cells or antigen-presenting cells move to lymph nodes causing a systemic sensitization and the development of asthma. Additional studies are needed to confirm this model in humans.

REFERENCES

1. Epidemiology in Wikipedia, 2009. Available at: http://en.wikipedia.org/wiki/Epidemiology. Accessed January 10, 2010.
2. Asher MI, Keil U, Anderson HR, et al. International Study of Asthma and Allergies in Childhood (ISAAC): rationale and methods. Eur Respir J 1995;8:483–91.
3. Pearce N, Weiland S, Keil U, et al. Self-reported prevalence of asthma symptoms in children in Australia, England, Germany and New Zealand: an international comparison using the ISAAC protocol. Eur Respir J 1993;6:1455–61.
4. Weiland S, Björkstén B, Brunekreef B, et al. Phase II of the International Study of Asthma and Allergies in Childhood (ISAAC II): rationale and methods. Eur Respir J 2004;24:406–12.
5. Worldwide variation in prevalence of symptoms of asthma, allergic rhinoconjunctivitis, and atopic eczema: ISAAC. The International Study of Asthma and Allergies in Childhood (ISAAC) Steering Committee. Lancet 1998;351:1225–32.

6. Asher MI, Montefort S, Bjorksten B, et al. Worldwide time trends in the prevalence of symptoms of asthma, allergic rhinoconjunctivitis, and eczema in childhood: ISAAC phases one and three repeat multicountry cross-sectional surveys. Lancet 2006;368:733–43.
7. Williams H, Stewart A, von Mutius E, et al. Is eczema really on the increase worldwide? J Allergy Clin Immunol 2008;121:947–54, e15.
8. Laughter D, Istvan JA, Tofte SJ, et al. The prevalence of atopic dermatitis in Oregon schoolchildren. J Am Acad Dermatol 2000;43:649–55.
9. Hanifin JM, Reed ML. A population-based survey of eczema prevalence in the United States. Dermatitis 2007;18:82–91.
10. Ricci G, Patrizi A, Baldi E, et al. Long-term follow-up of atopic dermatitis: retrospective analysis of related risk factors and association with concomitant allergic diseases. J Am Acad Dermatol 2006;55:765–71.
11. Illi S, von Mutius E, Lau S, et al. The natural course of atopic dermatitis from birth to age 7 years and the association with asthma. J Allergy Clin Immunol 2004;113: 925–31.
12. Perkin MR, Strachan DP, Williams HC, et al. Natural history of atopic dermatitis and its relationship to serum total immunoglobulin E in a population-based birth cohort study. Pediatr Allergy Immunol 2004;15:221–9.
13. Barnetson RS, Rogers M. Childhood atopic eczema. BMJ 2002;324:1376–9.
14. Martinez FD, Wright AL, Taussig LM, et al. Asthma and wheezing in the first six years of life. The Group Health Medical Associates. N Engl J Med 1995;332: 133–8.
15. Kulig M, Bergmann R, Klettke U, et al. Natural course of sensitization to food and inhalant allergens during the first 6 years of life. J Allergy Clin Immunol 1999;103: 1173–9.
16. Illi S, von Mutius E, Lau S, et al. The pattern of atopic sensitization is associated with the development of asthma in childhood. J Allergy Clin Immunol 2001;108: 709–14.
17. Gustafsson D, Sjöberg O, Foucard T. Development of allergies and asthma in infants and young children with atopic dermatitis–a prospective follow-up to 7 years of age. Allergy 2000;55:240–5.
18. Novembre E, Cianferoni A, Lombardi E, et al. Natural history of "intrinsic" atopic dermatitis. Allergy 2001;56:452–3.
19. Ohshima Y, Yamada A, Hiraoka M, et al. Early sensitization to house dust mite is a major risk factor for subsequent development of bronchial asthma in Japanese infants with atopic dermatitis: results of a 4-year followup study. Ann Allergy Asthma Immunol 2002;89:265–70.
20. Wuthrich B, Schmid-Grendelmeier P. Natural course of AEDS. Allergy 2002;57: 267–8.
21. van der Hulst AE, Klip H, Brand PL. Risk of developing asthma in young children with atopic eczema: a systematic review. J Allergy Clin Immunol 2007; 120:565–9.
22. Kapoor R, Menon C, Hoffstad O, et al. The prevalence of atopic triad in children with physician-confirmed atopic dermatitis. J Am Acad Dermatol 2008;58:68–73.
23. Stern DA, Morgan WJ, Halonen M, et al. Wheezing and bronchial hyperresponsiveness in early childhood as predictors of newly diagnosed asthma in early adulthood: a longitudinal birth-cohort study. Lancet 2008;372:1058–64.
24. Guilbert TW, Morgan WJ, Zeiger RS, et al. Atopic characteristics of children with recurrent wheezing at high risk for the development of childhood asthma. J Allergy Clin Immunol 2004;114:1282–7.

25. Lowe L, Murray CS, Custovic A, et al. Specific airway resistance in 3-year-old children: a prospective cohort study. Lancet 2002;359:1904–8.
26. Ker J, Hartert TV. The atopic march: what's the evidence? Ann Allergy Asthma Immunol 2009;103:282–9.
27. Cork MJ, Robinson DA, Vasilopoulos Y, et al. New perspectives on epidermal barrier dysfunction in atopic dermatitis: gene–environment interactions. J Allergy Clin Immunol 2006;118:3–21.
28. Seidenari S, Giusti G. Objective assessment of the skin of children affected by atopic dermatitis: a study of pH, capacitance and TEWL in eczematous and clinically uninvolved skin. Acta Derm Venereol 1995;75:429–33.
29. Akei HS, Brandt EB, Mishra A, et al. Epicutaneous aeroallergen exposure induces systemic TH2 immunity that predisposes to allergic nasal responses. J Allergy Clin Immunol 2006;118:62–9.
30. Lee GR, Flavell RA. Transgenic mice which overproduce Th2 cytokines develop spontaneous atopic dermatitis and asthma. Int Immunol 2004;16:1155–60.
31. Spergel JM, Mizoguchi E, Brewer JP, et al. Epicutaneous sensitization with protein antigen induces localized allergic dermatitis and hyperresponsiveness to methacholine after single exposure to aerosolized antigen in mice. J Clin Invest 1998;101:1614–22.
32. Spergel JM, Mizoguchi E, Oettgen H, et al. Roles of TH1 and TH2 cytokines in a murine model of allergic dermatitis. J Clin Invest 1999;103:1103–11.
33. Woodward AL, Spergel JM, Alenius H, et al. An obligate role for T-cell receptor alphabeta+ T cells but not T-cell receptor gammadelta+ T cells, B cells, or CD40/CD40L interactions in a mouse model of atopic dermatitis. J Allergy Clin Immunol 2001;107:359–66.
34. He R, Oyoshi MK, Garibyan L, et al. TSLP acts on infiltrating effector T cells to drive allergic skin inflammation. Proc Natl Acad Sci U S A 2008;105: 11875–80.
35. Demehri S, Morimoto M, Holtzman MJ, et al. Skin-derived TSLP triggers progression from epidermal-barrier defects to asthma. PLoS Biol 2009;7:e1000067.
36. He R, Oyoshi MK, Jin H, et al. Epicutaneous antigen exposure induces a Th17 response that drives airway inflammation after inhalation challenge. Proc Natl Acad Sci U S A 2007;104:15817–22.
37. Palmer CN, Irvine AD, Terron-Kwiatkowski A, et al. Common loss-of-function variants of the epidermal barrier protein filaggrin are a major predisposing factor for atopic dermatitis. Nat Genet 2006;38:441–6.
38. Hanifin JM. Evolving concepts of pathogenesis in atopic dermatitis and other eczemas. J Invest Dermatol 2009;129:320–2.
39. Kezic S, Kemperman PM, Koster ES, et al. Loss-of-function mutations in the filaggrin gene lead to reduced level of natural moisturizing factor in the stratum corneum. J Invest Dermatol 2008;128:2117–9.
40. Hudson TJ. Skin barrier function and allergic risk. Nat Genet 2006;38:399–400.
41. Smith FJ, Irvine AD, Terron-Kwiatkowski A, et al. Loss-of-function mutations in the gene encoding filaggrin cause ichthyosis vulgaris. Nat Genet 2006;38: 337–42.
42. Baurecht H, Irvine AD, Novak N, et al. Toward a major risk factor for atopic eczema: meta-analysis of filaggrin polymorphism data. J Allergy Clin Immunol 2007;120:1406–12.
43. Weidinger S, Illig T, Baurecht H, et al. Loss-of-function variations within the filaggrin gene predispose for atopic dermatitis with allergic sensitizations. J Allergy Clin Immunol 2006;118:214–9.

44. Barker JN, Palmer CN, Zhao Y, et al. Null mutations in the filaggrin gene (FLG) determine major susceptibility to early-onset atopic dermatitis that persists into adulthood. J Invest Dermatol 2007;127:564–7.
45. Weidinger S, O'Sullivan M, Illig T, et al. Filaggrin mutations, atopic eczema, hay fever, and asthma in children. J Allergy Clin Immunol 2008;121:1203–9, e1.
46. Ong PY, Ohtake T, Brandt C, et al. Endogenous antimicrobial peptides and skin infections in atopic dermatitis. N Engl J Med 2002;347:1151–60.
47. Castro-Rodriguez JA, Holberg CJ, Wright AL, et al. A clinical index to define risk of asthma in young children with recurrent wheezing. Am J Respir Crit Care Med 2000;162:1403–6.
48. Porsbjerg C, von Linstow ML, Ulrik CS, et al. Risk factors for onset of asthma: a 12-year prospective follow-up study. Chest 2006;129:309–16.

Quality-of-life Outcomes and Measurement in Childhood Atopic Dermatitis

Sarah L. Chamlin, MD[a,b,*], Mary-Margaret Chren, MD[c]

KEYWORDS

- Atopic dermatitis • Quality of life • Pediatric

Atopic dermatitis (AD) is the most common skin disease in children, affecting 7% to 17% of children in the United States.[1] Most children with AD develop the disease in the first 5 years of life, a critical time for physical and psychosocial development (see also the article by Jonathan M. Spergel elsewhere in this issue for further exploration of this topic). For example, children establish behavior and sleep patterns early in life, and AD may disrupt the establishment of normal sleep patterns, behavior, and relationships. Such physiologic and psychological effects, which not only change the life of the affected child but also affect the physical, social, and emotional functioning of parents, have been reported in young children with AD.[2] Several quality-of-life instruments have been developed to quantify this multidimensional effect on children and their families.[3–11] Such measures of the burden of AD can be used to improve the lives of afflicted children and their families.

BEHAVIOR AND EMOTIONS IN AD

AD affects the emotions and behavior of children, and these effects differ with the age of the child. Reported emotional symptoms for the young child with AD include irritability, fussiness, and increased crying, and parents most often attribute these

Supported by the National Institute of Arthritis Musculoskeletal and Skin Diseases (grant K24 AR 052667 to MMC).

[a] Division of Pediatric Dermatology, Children's Memorial Hospital, 2300 Children's Plaza, Box 107, Chicago, IL 60614, USA
[b] Department of Dermatology, Northwestern's Feinberg School of Medicine, Chicago, IL, USA
[c] Department of Dermatology, University of California at San Francisco, 4150 Clement Street 151R, San Francisco, CA 94121, USA
* Corresponding author. Children's Memorial Hospital, 2300 Children's Plaza, Box 107, Chicago, IL 60614.
E-mail address: schamlin@childrensmemorial.org

emotions to the symptom of pruritus.[2] In addition, parents of young children with AD describe their children as being more clingy, fearful, frustrated, and wanting to be held more.[2,12] Several studies have documented increasing psychological disturbances with increasing disease severity (see also the article by Kelsay and colleagues elsewhere in this issue for further exploration of this topic).[12,13]

Increased behavior and discipline problems have been documented and are increased in young children with AD, including excessive dependency, hyperactivity, restlessness, and scratching to get attention. Despite this increase, few studies have formally evaluated children with AD for attention-deficit/hyperactivity disorder (ADHD).[14–17] One report documented increased attention problems, disruptive behaviors, restlessness, and emotional sensitivity in children with AD.[14] More recently, a population-based study was published comparing the prevalence of ADHD in children with AD with a control group. A significant association between ADHD and AD was found.[17]

Few studies describe the emotional effects of AD on adolescents. Adolescence is a critical time for the development of self-identity and self-esteem,[18] and looking different as a result of skin disease can adversely affect teenagers during this important developmental stage. Adolescents and adults with acne vulgaris report increased anxiety, embarrassment, interpersonal difficulties, social isolation, shame, and self-consciousness, and adolescents affected by AD likely have similar or greater emotional effects because of their skin disease.[18–20] During validation, Skindex-teen, a 21-item quality-of-life scale specifically for adolescents with skin disease, was administered to 205 participants aged 12 to 18 years, 33 of whom had AD. The mean score for the group with AD was higher (indicating greater quality-of-life impairment) than the mean score for the groups with all other skin diseases (Aimee Smidt, MD, Albuquerque, NM, personal communication, October 9, 2009).

SLEEP, ITCH, AND AD

Although up to 30% of children experience sleep difficulties in the first few years of life,[21] sleep abnormalities are more prevalent in children with AD. Documented sleep dysfunctions include delayed onset of sleep, multiple awakenings, and an overall reduced sleep efficiency.[22–26] Sleep disturbance from pruritus and the subsequent reduced sleep efficiency often affects daytime behavior and productivity for the affected children.[22] Sleep abnormalities in school-aged children with AD have been studied with home polysomnography, a recording of overnight sleep physiology. Polysomnography revealed frequent awakenings associated with scratching episodes and an overall reduced sleep efficiency.[25] Awakenings persist for many children during disease remission and are often unassociated with scratching.[24] The cause of awakenings during disease remission is not known, but it is hypothesized that the sleep abnormality induced by pruritus may become a learned sleep pattern. Children with AD may associate sleep with itching, and scratching behavior may influence the development of an abnormal chronic behavior-based sleep pattern with frequent awakenings (see also the article by Kelsay and colleagues elsewhere in this issue for further exploration of this topic).

Sleep problems from any cause in infancy and early childhood have consequences, including greater difficulty awakening, daytime tiredness, and irritability, and may even be associated with a higher rate of ADHD.[27] Moreover, children with AD have documented difficulty falling asleep and night waking, which correlate with daytime behavior and discipline problems.[22] Daytime sleepiness is difficult to evaluate, and children with chronic sleep loss are often mistakenly misdiagnosed with behavioral abnormalities and learning disabilities.[22,26] Further work is needed on the cause-and-effect relationship of sleep abnormalities and behavioral issues in children with AD.

Cosleeping or bed sharing is a strategy documented in the parents of children with AD likely adopted to improve the sleep of their children, but cosleeping often leads to sleep deprivation for one or both parents.[2,28] Although cosleeping is common (12.8% in the United States[29] and even more prevalent in many cultures[30]) this sleep behavior is increased to 30% in families of young children with AD in the United States.[28] Parents of children with AD report bringing the child into their bed to prevent awakenings, and holding their child's hands to prevent scratching. This practice likely decreases the quality of the parents' sleep, leading to parental sleep deprivation and exhaustion.[23] If cosleeping behavior becomes habitual for children and their families, this practice may perpetuate the child's sleep disturbance beyond the time of disease flare. Sleep disturbances and cosleeping in children with AD and their parents are directly associated with severity of AD, and likely correlate with overall decreased quality of life.[28]

THE EFFECT OF AD ON THE FAMILY

In addition to the effects on the child, childhood AD can affect the emotional, financial, physical, and social well-being of parents.[31,32] Mothers of young children with AD report poor social support, decreased employment outside the home, stress about parenting, and difficulty with discipline.[12] In addition, increased AD disease severity is strongly associated with a greater effect on the family, which decreases as disease severity lessens, highlighting the importance of understanding and measuring the burden of disease on the entire family.[33–36] The effect on the family is increased when parents perceive high disease severity, worry about payment for medical care, and seek nonmedical or over-the-counter products therapy.[32] It is not uncommon for parents of a child with AD to change their lifestyle and home environment dramatically to help cope with the needs of their atopic child. These changes may be financially burdensome and stressful and include changes in their homes (flooring, heating, and air-conditioning systems), vacations, and activities. In addition, parents complain of exhaustion and fatigue, likely as a result of sleep deprivation. Parent sleep deprivation can be notable, and the mean sleep loss was quantified in one study as 1.9 hours and 1.5 hours for the severe and moderate disease groups, respectively.[37] Another study noted 39 minutes of sleep loss for mothers and 45 minutes of loss for fathers, and severity of sleep disturbance was correlated with maternal anxiety and depression.[38]

Parents of children with AD have many worries, including triggers for disease flares (ie, diet and environment), the cause of disease, costs of care, proper use of medications, and long-term outcomes for their child's health, well-being, and self-esteem.[2] In addition, parents commonly worry about and fear the use and side effects of topical corticosteroids. In a questionnaire-based study, 72.5% participants worried about using topical steroids on their own or their child's skin. This worry led to noncompliance in 24% of individuals.[39] In the International Study of Life with Atopic Eczema (ISOLATE), patients and caregivers reported delaying use of topical steroids for approximately 1 week after onset of a flare.[40] This study highlights parental response to fear of medication use, with suboptimal adherence, undertreatment of disease, and the desire to seek alternative therapies, some of which may be unproven, unbeneficial, or harmful.

Parents also report significant emotional effects, including sadness, crying, guilt, and self-blame, as a result of having a child with AD. They may blame themselves because they had or have atopic disease, or they may blame their atopic spouse for their child's illness. Parents often feel responsible for exposing their children to food or environmental allergens that they believe cause or worsen the dermatitis. In addition, negative reactions of friends, relatives, and the public can be emotionally stressful for parents and often evoke feelings of anger, sadness, helplessness, embarrassment, frustration, and disappointment. Moreover, parents report accusations of child abuse or neglect from strangers and the offering of unsolicited advice as a common occurrence. To avoid such conflict, parents of children with AD may stay home more to avoid these negative interactions and thus may develop feeling of social isolation.[2]

MEASURING QUALITY-OF-LIFE AND EFFECT OF AD ON THE FAMILY

Quality of life is defined broadly as an individual's well-being. More precisely, health-related quality of life is an outcome that extends beyond traditional views of mortality and morbidity and includes the health dimensions of symptoms, the functional effect of disease, and the broad psychological, social, and emotional effect of disease.[41] For pediatric patients, quality of life is relevant for the affected child as well as the parents and siblings. To measure quality of life in young children and infants, parents are often asked to answer questions as a proxy for their children.

Quality-of-life measurement scales for use in pediatrics are generic or disease specific and many are age specific. Each type has a different application. For example, generic instruments are useful for comparing the effects of different diseases on children. Such a comparison was made using a generic instrument, the family questionnaire of Stein and Reissman, to compare the effect on the family of childhood AD with juvenile-onset diabetes mellitus. The investigators reported that families of children with moderate to severe AD were affected to a greater degree compared with families of diabetic children.[37] The lack of support for families struggling with AD compared with the support offered to families of diabetic children was suggested as a possible explanation. Another study used the Children's Life Quality Index, a skin disease–specific scale, to compare children with skin disease including AD with other childhood diseases. The greatest effect measured was for cerebral palsy followed by generalized AD, renal disease, and cystic fibrosis.[42]

A few skin-specific quality-of-life scales have been developed for children and teenagers with skin disease. One such measure is the Children's Dermatology Life Quality Index (CDLQI), which was developed to measure the effects of skin disease on children from 3 to 16 years of age. With the initial validation of this scale, the greatest quality-of-life effects were on children with scabies and eczema.[3] This finding intuitively makes sense, with diseases with greater symptomatology (itch in both cases) having a higher effect on quality of life. A more recent study using the CDLQI reported the greatest quality-of-life effect on children with psoriasis, generalized eczema, and urticaria.[42] A cartoon version and several foreign-language translations of the CDLQI have been developed and published.[6]

When the secondary effect of skin disease, the family effect, is used to compare the effect of different diseases similar results are reported. The Family Dermatology Life Quality Index, another skin disease–specific scale, was used to compare the effect of different skin diseases on families. The greatest effect was seen with inflammatory skin disease and more specifically with eczema, psoriasis, and acne than all other skin diseases.[9]

Disease-specific quality-of-life scales for children with AD have been developed and are used as more sensitive and comprehensive measures of the specific effects of the disease. Disease-specific quality-of-life measures for children with AD include the Dermatitis Family Impact questionnaire (DFI),[4] the Infants' Dermatitis Quality of Life

Index (IDQOL),[5] the Childhood Atopic Dermatitis Impact Scale (CADIS),[7] the Parents' Index of Quality of life in Atopic Dermatitis (PIQoL-AD),[8] the Childhood Impact of Atopic Dermatitis,[10] and the Quality of Life in Primary Caregivers of Children with Atopic Dermatitis.[11] The reliability and validity for most of these instruments have been evaluated and published. Measurement of quality of life with these scales has been performed primarily in clinical research, including pharmaceutical trials, but their usefulness has not been shown in daily and routine clinical practice. Each scale may be advantageous in different situations. For example, the brief 10-item DFI and IDQOL measure primarily symptoms and functioning and can be completed in a few minutes.[4,5] The longer 45-item CADIS and 28-item PIQol-AD weigh the emotional effects of disease more heavily, but take longer to complete.[7,8]

DECREASING THE BURDEN OF DISEASE

It is likely that existing systems of care for children with AD are not adequate to support the emotional and social needs of many children with AD and their families.[37] Because of the multifaceted nature of the disease and its effects on patients and their families, support groups, detailed educational sessions, and specialty clinics are feasible methods to improve quality of life in this population.[33–36] However, some families and children with severe psychosocial dysfunction may require additional care such as professional psychiatric intervention.

Although support groups for pediatric patients and their families are believed to be beneficial, few data support this widely held belief.[43–46] Support groups may help families develop positive coping strategies, increase compliance with treatment, and diminish feelings of isolation, and many practitioners recognize these unproven benefits. The National Eczema Association is one such support group for patients with AD and their families (http://www.nationaleczema.org). One published study examined the effects of support groups and education on children with AD and their families using the CDLQI and an itch scale. The CDLQI scores in the intervention group significantly improved in this preliminary study, suggesting a positive role for disease-specific support groups and education.[47]

In addition to support groups, structured education, and specialty care from AD specialists, including dermatologists, pediatric dermatologists, allergist-immunologists, and dermatology nurses, may decrease the burden of disease and improve quality of life for children with AD and their parents.[48–57] Nurse educators may play a critical role in this process. For example, most parents are never shown how to apply topical treatments and most often apply less than indicated and less frequently than prescribed. Following repeated education and demonstration of application of topical steroids and emollients, disease severity dramatically decreased in a study of 51 children with poorly controlled AD.[48] Another study reported a decreased effect on the family when care was received from a dermatologist in an academic medical center.[49] In addition, satisfaction with care may even be increased when a specialized nurse practitioner is involved in the education and management.[53]

Although access to AD specialists and financial support for nurse practitioners and educators may be limited, specialty care and intensive education may ultimately be cost effective in children with moderate and severe AD.

SUMMARY

AD often affects the emotional and psychosocial functioning of afflicted children and their families. Children and families must cope with the physical symptoms, complex emotional effects, lifestyle changes, and social limitations imposed by this disease.

Not only is treatment of the dermatitis indicated, but if childhood behavioral, emotional, or sleep abnormalities are noted, these should be addressed early, when intervention may be more effective. The effect on the family can be measured and most often improves as disease severity improves. Improved education and support for children with AD and their families may improve quality of life.

REFERENCES

1. Laughter D, Istvan JA, Tofte SJ, et al. The prevalence of atopic dermatitis in Oregon schoolchildren. J Am Acad Dermatol 2000;43:649–55.
2. Chamlin SL, Frieden IJ, Williams ML, et al. The effects of atopic dermatitis on young American children and their families. Pediatrics 2004;114:607–11.
3. Lewis-Jones MS, Finlay AY. The Children's Dermatology Life Quality Index: initial validation and practical use. Br J Dermatol 1995;132:942–9.
4. Lawson V, Lewis-Jones MS, Finlay AY, et al. The family impact of childhood atopic dermatitis: the Dermatitis Family Impact questionnaire. Br J Dermatol 1998;138:107–13.
5. Lewis-Jones MS, Finlay AY, Dykes PJ. The infant's dermatitis quality of life index. Br J Dermatol 2001;144:104–10.
6. Holme SA, Man JL, Sharpe JL, et al. The Children's Dermatology Life Quality Index: validation of the cartoon version. Br J Dermatol 2003;148:285–90.
7. Chamlin SL, Cella D, Frieden IJ, et al. Validity of the Childhood Atopic Dermatitis Impact Scale (CADIS): a quality-of-life measure for young children with atopic dermatitis and their families. J Invest Dermatol 2005;125:1106–11.
8. McKenna SP, Whalley D, Dewar AL, et al. International development of the Parents' Index of Quality of Life in Atopic Dermatitis (PIQoL). Qual Life Res 2005;14:231–41.
9. Basra MKA, Sue-Ho R, Finlay AY. The Family Dermatology Life Quality Index: measuring the secondary impact of skin disease. Br J Dermatol 2007;156:528–38.
10. McKenna SP, Doward LC, Meads DM, et al. Quality of life in infants and children with atopic dermatitis: addressing issues of differential item functioning across countries in multinational clinical trials. Health Qual Life Outcomes 2007;5:45–52.
11. Kondo-Endo K, Ohashi Y, Nakagawa H, et al. Development and validation of a questionnaire measuring Quality of Life in Primary Caregivers of Children with Atopic Dermatitis (QPCAD). Br J Dermatol 2009;161:617–25.
12. Daud LR, Garralda ME, David TJ. Psychosocial adjustment in preschool children with atopic eczema. Arch Dis Child 1993;69:670–6.
13. Absolon CM, Cottrell D, Eldridge SM, et al. Psychological disturbance in atopic eczema: the extent of the problem in school-aged children. Br J Dermatol 1997;137:241–5.
14. Roth N, Beyreiss J, Schlenzka K, et al. Coincidence of attention deficit disorder and atopic disorders in children: empirical findings and hypothetical background. J Abnorm Child Psychol 1991;19:1–12.
15. Pelsser LMJ, Buitelaar JK, Savelkoul HFJ. ADHD as a (non) allergic hypersensitivity disorder: a hypothesis. Pediatr Allergy Immunol 2009;20:107–12.
16. Schmitt J, Romanos M. Lack of studies investigating the association of childhood eczema, sleeping problems, and attention-deficit/hyperactivity disorder. Pediatr Allergy Immunol 2009;20:299–300.
17. Schmitt J, Romanos M, Schmitt NM, et al. Atopic eczema and attention-deficit/hyperactivity disorder in a population-based sample of children and adolescents. JAMA 2009;301:724–6.

18. Smith JA. The impact of skin disease on the quality of life of adolescents. Adolesc Med State Art Rev 2001;12(2):343–53.
19. Krowchuk DP, Stancin T, Keskinen R, et al. The psychosocial effects of acne on adolescents. Pediatr Dermatol 1991;8(4):332–8.
20. Wu SF, Kinder BN, Trunnell TN, et al. Role of anxiety and anger in acne patients: a relationship with the severity of the disorder. J Am Acad Dermatol 1988;18: 325–33.
21. Johnson M. Infant and toddler sleep: a telephone survey of parents in one community. J Dev Behav Pediatr 1991;12:108–14.
22. Dahl RE, Bernhisel-Broadbent J, Scanlon-Holdford S, et al. Sleep disturbances in children with atopic dermatitis. Arch Pediatr Adolesc Med 1995;149:856–60.
23. Reid P, Lewis-Jones MS. Sleep difficulties and their management in preschoolers with atopic eczema. Clin Exp Dermatol 1995;20:38–41.
24. Reuveni H, Chapnick G, Tal A, et al. Sleep fragmentation in children with atopic dermatitis. Arch Pediatr Adolesc Med 1999;153:249–53.
25. Stores G, Burrows A, Crawford C. Physiological sleep disturbance in children with atopic dermatitis: a case control study. Pediatr Dermatol 1998;15:264–8.
26. Moldofsky H. Evaluation of daytime sleepiness. Clin Chest Med 1992;3:417–25.
27. Thunstrom M. Severe sleep problems in infancy associated with subsequent development of attention-deficit/hyperactivity disorder at 5.5 years of age. Acta Paediatr 2002;91:584–92.
28. Chamlin SL, Mattson CL, Frieden IJ, et al. The price of pruritus: sleep disturbance and co-sleeping in atopic dermatitis. Arch Pediatr Adolesc Med 2005;159:745–50.
29. Willinger M, Chia-Wen K, Hoffman HJ, et al. Trends in infant bed sharing in the United States, 1993–2000. Arch Pediatr Adolesc Med 2003;157:43–9.
30. Nelson EA, Taylor BJ, ICCPS Study Group. International care practices study: infant sleeping environment. Early Hum Dev 2001;62:43–55.
31. Warschburger P, Buchholz HT, Petermann F. Psychological adjustment in parents of young children with atopic dermatitis: which factors predict parental quality of life? Br J Dermatol 2004;150:304–11.
32. Balkrishnan R, Housman TS, Grummer S, et al. The family impact of atopic dermatitis in children: the role of the parent caregiver. Pediatr Dermatol 2003; 20(1):5–10.
33. Ben-Gashir MA, Seed PT, Hay RJ. Are quality of family life and disease severity related in childhood atopic dermatitis? J Eur Acad Dermatol Venereol 2002;16: 455–62.
34. Balkrishnan R, Housman TS, Carroll C, et al. Disease severity and associated family impact in childhood atopic dermatitis. Arch Dis Child 2003;88:423–7.
35. Aziah MSN, Rosnah T, Mardziah A, et al. Childhood atopic dermatitis: a measurement of quality of life and family impact. Med J Malaysia 2002;57:329–39.
36. Ben-Gashir MA, Seed PT, Hay RJ. Quality of life and disease severity are correlated in children with atopic dermatitis. Br J Dermatol 2004;150:284–90.
37. Su JC, Kemp AS, Varigos GA, et al. Atopic eczema: its impact on the family and financial cost. Arch Dis Child 1997;76:159–62.
38. Moore K, David TJ, Murray F, et al. Effect of childhood eczema and asthma on parental sleep and well-being: a prospective comparative study. Br J Dermatol 2006;154:514–8.
39. Charman CR, Morris AD, Williams HC. Topical corticosteroid phobia in patients with atopic eczema. Br J Dermatol 2000;142:931–6.
40. Zuberbier T, Orlow SJ, Paller AS, et al. Patient perspectives on the management of atopic dermatitis. J Allergy Clin Immunol 2006;118:226–32.

41. VanBeek M, Beach S, Braslow JB, et al. Highlights from the report of the working group on "core measure of the burden of skin disease". J Invest Dermatol 2007; 127:2701–6.

42. Beattie PE, Lewis-Jones MS. A comparative study of impairment of quality of life in children with skin disease and children with other chronic childhood diseases. Br J Dermatol 2006;155:145–51.

43. Harris H. Support groups: great for patients, great for your practice. Med Econ 1988;65:118–29.

44. Plante WA, Lobato D, Engel R. Review of group interventions for pediatric chronic conditions. J Pediatr Psychol 2001;26:435–53.

45. Epstein I, Stinson J, Stevens B. The effects of camp on health-related quality of life in children with chronic illnesses: a review of the literature. J Pediatr Oncol Nurs 2005;22:89–103.

46. Ersser SJ, Latter S, Sibley A, et al. Psychological and educational interventions for atopic eczema in children. Cochrane Database Syst Rev 2007;(18):CD004054.

47. Weber MB, de Tarso da Luz Fontes Neto P, Prati C, et al. Improvement of pruritus and quality of life of children with atopic dermatitis and their families after joining support groups. J Eur Acad Dermatol Venereol 2008;22:992–7.

48. Cork MJ, Britton J, Butler L, et al. Comparison of parent knowledge, therapy utilization and severity of atopic eczema before and after explanation and demonstration of topical therapies by a specialist dermatology nurse. Br J Dermatol 2003;149:582–9.

49. Balkrishnan R, Manuel J, Clarke J, et al. Effects of an episode of specialist care on the impact of childhood atopic dermatitis on the child's family. J Pediatr Health Care 2003;17(4):184–9.

50. Chinn DJ, Poyner T, Sibley G. Randomized controlled trial of a single dermatology nurse consultation in primary care on the quality of life of children with atopic eczema. Br J Dermatol 2002;146:432–9.

51. Staab D, von Rueden U, Kehrt R, et al. Evaluation of a parental training program for the management of childhood atopic dermatitis. Pediatr Allergy Immunol 2002;13:84–90.

52. Moore E, Williams A, Manias E, et al. Nurse-led clinics reduce severity of childhood atopic eczema: a review of the literature. Br J Dermatol 2006;155:1242–8.

53. Schuttelaar MLA, Vermeulen KM, Drukker N, et al. A randomized controlled trial in children with eczema: nurse practitioner vs. dermatologist. Br J Dermatol 2010; 162:162–70.

54. Beattie PE, Lewis-Jones MS. An audit of the impact of a consultation with a paediatric dermatology team on quality of life in infants with atopic eczema and their families: further validation of the Infants' Dermatitis Quality of Life Index and Dermatitis Family Impact score. Br J Dermatol 2006;155:1249–55.

55. Moore EJ, Williams A, Manias E, et al. Eczema workshops reduce severity of childhood atopic eczema. Australas J Dermatol 2009;50:100–6.

56. Ricci G, Bendandi B, Aiazzi R, et al. Three years of Italian experience of an educational program for parents of young children affected by atopic dermatitis: improving knowledge produces lower anxiety levels in parents of children with atopic dermatitis. Pediatr Dermatol 2009;26:1–5.

57. Grillo M, Gassner L, Marshman G, et al. Pediatric atopic eczema: the impact of an educational intervention. Pediatr Dermatol 2006;23:428–36.

Allergic Triggers in Atopic Dermatitis

Jean-Christoph Caubet, MD[a,b,c], Philippe A. Eigenmann, MD[a,b],*

KEYWORDS

- Atopic dermatitis • Eczema • Allergic trigger
- Food • Aeroallergens

Atopic dermatitis (AD) is an inflammatory, chronically relapsing, and intensely pruritic skin disease. Numerous names have been used for this most frequent inflammatory disease in childhood, reflecting different approaches and definitions. The local inflammation of the skin has always been described as dermatitis. The term "eczema" has been suggested to describe a variety of skin diseases with common clinical characteristics, all involving a genetically determined skin barrier defect.[1] In children and young adults with atopy, the underlying inflammation is dominated by high serum IgE levels and IgE-antibody–associated reactions, which allows use of the term atopic eczema or AD. This terminology suggests a potential role for allergens as triggers in this disease.

AD affects a large number of children and adults in industrialized countries. More than 10% of all children are affected at some time during childhood.[2] The onset of AD occurs during the first 6 months of life in 45% of children, during the first year of life in 60% and before the age of 5 years in at least 85% of affected individuals.[3] Patients with severe AD and early sensitization to allergens typically have a persisting illness, sometimes lasting for a lifetime. Childhood AD can be a very disabling disease with an important impact on the quality of life of the children and their parents (see the article by Chamlin and Chren elsewhere in this issue for further exploration of this topic).

Nonatopic dermatitis (non-IgE mediated) is more common in preschool children and adults. Studies have shown a prevalence of 45% to 64% in children,[4,5] but even in adults, figures as high as 40% have been reported.[6] Nonatopic children with eczema have been reported to have a lower risk of developing asthma than atopic children with eczema. It is noteworthy that nonatopic dermatitis in children may evolve into AD.

This review focuses on AD, which by definition is associated with elevated IgE. The authors define the role of allergens in the pathogenesis of AD, comment on the various

[a] University Hospitals of Geneva, Geneva, Switzerland
[b] University of Geneva Medical School, Geneva, Switzerland
[c] Division of Pediatric Allergy and Immunology, Mount Sinai School of Medicine, New York, NY, USA
* Corresponding author. Adult & Child Allergy Unit, 4, rue Gabrielle-Perret-Gentil, CH-1211 Genève 14, Switzerland.
E-mail address: Philippe.Eigenmann@hcuge.ch

Immunol Allergy Clin N Am 30 (2010) 289–307
doi:10.1016/j.iac.2010.06.002
0889-8561/10/$ – see front matter

potential allergen triggers of eczema, their clinical consequences, and the impact on diagnosis and treatment of AD.

ROLE OF ALLERGENS IN AD

AD is a paradigmatic skin disease that is the product of a complex interaction between various susceptibility genes, defects in skin barrier function, a specific immunologic response, and a clear interaction with infectious agents and the host environment (**Fig. 1**).[7] Although the exact mechanisms of the disease are still not fully elucidated, extensive research in recent years has shed light on the role of allergens in AD. At cellular and molecular levels, evidence strongly implicates an allergic component in AD, primarily in children. A multitude of allergens has been incriminated (**Table 1**), and the largest part of the studies have focused on food allergens. The role of aeroallergens has been investigated to a lesser extent, and is discussed in the second part of this article.

Genetically predisposed patients with AD have an epidermal barrier dysfunction mainly caused by decreased ceramide levels and loss of the function of filaggrin, which is a crucial protein in the cutaneous barrier function; this results mostly in enhanced transepidermal water loss.[8] In addition, the partial loss of the barrier function can facilitate the penetration of environmental allergens and promote allergic skin inflammation. Environmental allergens potentially include aeroallergens,[9] as well as in some cases food allergens.[10] A recent study showed that children who have never been exposed to peanut during the prenatal period and with negative tests for peanut-specific IgE in the cord blood were sensitized to peanut allergens as a result of application of skin preparations containing peanut oil on inflamed skin.[10] This result suggested that a primary sensitization to a food allergen occurred before ingestion of the implicated food through a route of sensitization other than the oral route.

For food allergens, sensitization occurs mostly via the gastrointestinal tract. The absorption of unaltered proteins into the circulation is a normal, physiologic phenomenon occurring in nonatopic as well as atopic individuals of all ages.[11,12] Similar to the altered skin barrier, gut barrier dysfunction might play a role in patients with AD and food allergy.[13,14] Studies have shown that patients with AD have a facilitated absorption resulting from IgE molecules present on gut epithelial cells, followed by increased

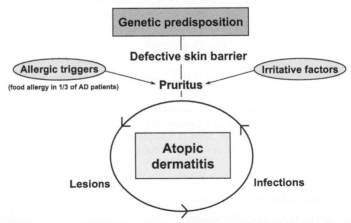

Fig. 1. Interaction of the different triggers incriminated in the pathogenesis of atopic dermatitis (AD).

Table 1		
Allergic triggers of AD		
Food Allergens	**Microorganisms**	**Aeroallergens**
Cow's milk	Bacteria	Pollen
Egg	*Staphylococcus aureus*	Mold
Soy	*Streptococcus species*	Dust mite
Wheat	Fungi	Animal dander
Peanut	*Trichophyton*	Cockroach
Tree nuts	*Malassezia*	
Fish	*Candida*	
Shellfish		

Data from Leung D. Pediatric allergy: principles and practice. St Louis: Mosby; 2003.

antigen transfer across the gut barrier. Rapidly absorbed food proteins circulate throughout the body, and can then initiate and perpetuate immune responses in the skin.

The immune response to an allergen in the skin of AD patients is complex and involves both IgE-mediated immediate immune responses and T-cell–mediated delayed immune responses.[15]

Many studies addressing the pathophysiology of AD have focused on serum IgE, with titers above the normal range in approximately 85% of patients with AD.[16] Approximately 85% of these patients have positive specific IgE antibodies to foods and inhalant allergens.[6,16,17] Receptors for IgE antibodies have been identified on dendritic cells, T cells, B cells, monocytes, macrophages, eosinophils, and platelets.[18–20]

Langerhans cells (LC), bearing allergen-specific IgE antibodies on their surface, are more numerous in AD lesions and appear to play an important role in cutaneous allergen presentation to T-helper 2 (Th2) cells. The LC-bound IgE facilitates capture and internalization of allergens prior to their processing and antigen presentation to T cells. Normal individuals and patients with respiratory allergy have low-level surface expression of FcεRI on their LC, whereas FcεRI is expressed at high levels in the inflammatory environment of AD. IgE-bearing LC are 100- to 1000-fold more efficient at presenting allergen to T cells (primarily Th2 cells) and activating T-cell proliferation.[21] After capture of the allergen, activated dendritic cells activate memory Th2 cells in atopic skin, but they may also migrate to the lymph nodes to stimulate naïve T cells to further expand the pool of systemic Th2 cells.

T lymphocytes play a key role in AD. This idea was initially supported by the observation that patients with primary T-cell immunodeficiency disorders frequently have increased serum IgE level and eczematous skin lesions, which clear after bone marrow grafting.[17,22] The observation was reinforced by the fact that eczematous rashes do not occur in the absence of T cells in animal models.[23] Food antigen–specific[24] and aeroallergen-specific[25] T cells have been cloned from active skin lesions and as well as from normal skin in patients with AD. Food antigen–specific T cells have been isolated in peripheral blood from individuals with relevant food protein–induced AD.[26–28] These specific cells express the cutaneous lymphocyte antigen (CLA), involved in the recruitment of allergen-specific T cells to the skin, which has not been observed in patients with other allergic diseases such as asthma or gastrointestinal allergies.[28,29]

In acute skin lesions, infiltrating T lymphocytes predominantly express Th2 cytokines, interleukin (IL)-4, and IL-13, whereas T cells in chronic lesions predominantly express IL-5 and IL-12. Hence, cytokines expressed in lesions of AD reflect the characteristics of a typical allergic milieu. Th2-type cytokines promote chronic allergic inflammation by up-regulating adhesion molecules on vascular endothelial cells including vascular cell adhesion molecule 1 (VCAM-1), E-selectin, and intercellular adhesion molecule 1 (ICAM-1),[30] by up-regulating high-affinity receptors for IgE antibodies on LC and other antigen-presenting cells through recruiting inflammatory cells to the site, and by promoting local production of IgE antibodies.[21,31] Adhesion molecules are not typically expressed in the skin of nonatopic individuals but are expressed in nonlesional skin of AD patients, and are markedly up-regulated in skin lesions or following epicutaneous application of allergens in sensitized AD patients.[32]

T regulatory cells have been described as a further subtype of T cells that can play a role in AD. This proposal is supported by the observation that patients with immune dysregulation, polyendrocrinopathy, enteropathy X-linked (IPEX) syndrome characterized by high IgE levels, food allergy, and eczematous lesions have mutations in FOXP3, a nuclear factor expressed in regulatory T cells.[33]

In addition to T cells, eosinophils have been implicated in the pathogenesis of AD. Although eosinophils are not prominent in histologic sections of AD lesions as in allergen-induced asthma, immunohistochemical staining of AD skin has revealed prominent deposits of the eosinophil major basic protein and eosinophil-derived neurotoxin in active eczematous lesions.[34,35] Major basic protein is a cytolytic protein secreted almost exclusively by eosinophils that is capable of damaging skin epithelial cells and promoting mast cell degranulation. These deposits are not found in uninvolved skin sites in AD patients.[36] The role of eosinophils was confirmed by oral food challenges (OFC) in food-allergic AD patients. A marked increase in plasma histamine concentrations,[37] activation of plasma eosinophils,[38] and infiltration of eosinophils and elaboration of eosinophil products in skin lesions were observed after the challenge test.[16,36,39] Eosinophils are part of the late phase response that was regulated by Th2 cytokines (IL-4, IL-5, IL-13) and eotaxin-1.[40,41] These studies provide further evidences of an allergic component in a subgroup of AD patients.

In comparison with patients with AD without food allergy or normal controls, children with AD and food hypersensitivity exposed to the relevant allergen were found to have high basophil histamine release in vitro.[42] When placed on an appropriate food allergen elimination diet for 1 year, the skin condition significantly improved and spontaneous basophil histamine release decreased. Peripheral blood mononuclear cells from food-allergic subjects with high spontaneous basophil histamine release were found to elaborate a 23-kDa cytokine called histamine-releasing factor (HRF) that can activate basophils from food-sensitive, but not food-tolerant, children.[43] Several isoforms of IgE are secreted, and it has been postulated that HRF interacts with specific isoforms of IgE.[44]

Microorganisms can also provide allergic triggers. Most patients with AD are colonized with *Staphylococcus aureus* and experience exacerbation of their skin disease after infection with this organism.[45] In this regard, IgE antibodies to *S aureus* exotoxins were found in close to 60% of patients with moderate to severe AD.[46] IgE to the exotoxins could not be detected in normal controls, patients with respiratory allergy, or patients with psoriasis. These exotoxins may contribute to the biphasic inflammatory response not only by allergen-specific activation of FcεRI-bearing effector cells but also in their capacity to act as superantigens by non-MHC restricted activation of large numbers of stimulated T cells.[46,47] In a similar way, IgE sensitization to *Malassezia* species is observed in patients with AD but not in those with asthma or allergic rhinitis without AD.[48,49]

AD is a complex disease involving barrier defects and chronic inflammation. As reviewed here, currently available data strongly suggest a major role for allergic triggers in AD at a cellular and molecular level.

AD AND FOOD ALLERGENS

The potential role of food allergens in AD has been long debated. As early as the beginning of the 1900s, several case reports showed an improvement of AD after avoiding specific food,[50] with reoccurrence of the lesions when the food was reintroduced. Thereafter, well-designed studies, mostly in the past two decades, clearly pointed to a pathogenic role for food hypersensitivity in a subset of children and adolescents with AD, as removal of the causative food led to improvement in skin symptoms,[51–55] introduction of the causative food provoked the disorder,[56–59] and avoidance of the causative food helped prevent the disorder.[60–62]

Prevalence of Food Allergy in Patients with AD

To provide an accurate diagnosis, the prevalence of food allergy in AD patients should be well defined in a given population. Similarly to other chronic atopic disorders such asthma, various triggers add to the difficulty of designing well-controlled prevalence studies. Nevertheless, several well-designed studies provide a good estimation of the prevalence of food allergy in AD. In westernized countries the prevalence of food allergy is estimated to be 6% to 8% in children and 2% to 3% in adults.[63] The prevalence rate is much higher in patients with AD, with age of the patient and severity of the AD both factors, as severe AD and younger age are risk factors for food allergy.[64] During the past 20 years, a large number of studies using double-blind placebo-controlled food challenges (DBPCFC) to support the role of foods as triggers of AD have been published (**Table 2**). Although the prevalence may vary between the studies, likely due to different methodology, approximately one-third of the patients with moderate to severe AD have food allergy as demonstrated by positive DBPCFC to selected food.[21] In one of the largest series supporting the link between food allergy and AD, Sicherer and Sampson[65] performed more than 2000 DBPCFC, out of which approximately 40% were positive.

Unfortunately, comparing these studies is difficult because of the various definitions used for positivity or the type of study (retrospective, prospective, or case-controlled

Table 2
Prevalence of food allergy in children with AD based on double-blind placebo-controlled food challenges[a]

Study	Years	N	Food Allergy (%)
Sampson et al	1985	113	56
Burks et al	1988	46	33
Sampson et al	1992	320	63
Eigenmann et al	1998	63	37
Burks et al	1998	165	39
Niggenmann et al	1999	107	51
Eigenmann et al	2000	74	34
Breuer et al	2004	64	46

[a] *Data from* Rance F, Boguniewicz M, Lau S. New visions for atopic eczema: An iPAC summary and future trends. Pediatr Allergy Immunol:2008;19:17–25.

studies). Another problem related to these studies is that the intensity of the eczema was not scored systematically before and on the day after the OFC, as late reactions might occur (on the day after the OFC or even later). Another point of controversy is related to a potential selection bias (patients referred to the allergist for possible food allergy), which may lead to a potential overestimation of the prevalence. When considering only the patients recruited through a dermatology clinic, the prevalence was slightly lower (27%).[66] Worthy of note is that most studies were performed in referral clinics, possibly leading to figures higher than the "true" prevalence.

In adults, studies with a sufficient number of patients to evaluate the prevalence are lacking, but most investigators agree that food hypersensitivity plays a very minor role in adult AD.[21,67,68] To support this, Woods and colleagues[69] reported that prevalence of food allergy in 41 randomly selected young adults was 1.3%. Japanese investigators found a much higher prevalence of food-induced eczema (44%), although the causative foods were uncommon allergens, including chocolate, coffee, and rice, suggesting nonallergic adverse effects of foods.[70]

Foods Triggering AD

Hen's egg, milk, wheat, soy, peanut, nuts, and fish are responsible for more than 90% of food allergy in AD patients.[65] The incriminated foods vary according to the age of the patients (**Table 3**). Besides the frequently incriminated "classical" food proteins, other food components can exacerbate AD in individual patients.[71] Whether these reactions are allergic or nonimmunologic "pseudoallergic" reactions is not yet clear.[72] Sugar as a suspected food trigger plays no role according to the results of oral challenge tests and is overestimated by many patients or their parents.[73]

Patients with birch pollen sensitization can also react on OFC with cross-reacting foods, with exacerbation of eczema.[74] Triggering of AD by pollen-associated food is especially relevant in adolescent and adult patients. In an unselected population the inducibility of eczema by pollen-associated food appears to be low.[75]

Patterns of Clinical Reactions to Food in AD Patients

Based on OFC, studies with large numbers of patients have shown that cutaneous reactions occurred in 74% of the tested patients with AD, and that isolated skin symptoms were observed in only 30% of reactions.[21] Skin reactions generally consisted of pruritic, morbilliform, or macular eruption appearing on predilection sites for AD (head,

Table 3
Foods more commonly involved in food allergy, according to age

Infants	Children (2–10 Years)	Adolescents and Young Adults
Cow's milk	Cow's milk	Peanut
Egg	Egg	Tree nuts
Wheat	Peanut	Fish
Soy	Tree nuts	Shellfish
	Fish	Sesame
	Shellfish	Pollen-associated foods
	Sesame	
	Kiwi fruit	

Data from Sampson HA. Update on food allergy. J Allergy Clin Immunol 2004;113:805–19.

neck, and creases). Gastrointestinal and respiratory symptoms were less frequent, occurring in approximately 50% and 45%, respectively.[21]

Food-induced reactions in AD may occur at various times after a positive OFC.[76]

Immediate IgE-mediated reactions occur mostly within 2 hours after ingesting food. DBPCFC clearly demonstrated an immediate IgE-mediated food hypersensitivity reaction in a subset of children with AD.[21,71,74] Such distinct food-induced symptoms are rarely seen during "natural exposure" to foods, as foods are generally not ingested on an empty stomach following prolonged periods of food allergen avoidance,[21] because repeated ingestion of a food allergen can result in a down-regulation of the immediate response.[77]

These children typically present with urticaria or angioedema as well as other immediate-type reactions involving the gastrointestinal or respiratory tracts, or less frequently with anaphylactic shock. Some patients may present with only pruritus within 2 hours after food ingestion, suggesting an IgE-mediated mechanism, with subsequent scratching leading to an AD exacerbation.

Isolated eczematous delayed reactions, that is, flares of eczema usually after 6 to 48 hours, are suggestive of a non-IgE–mediated reaction. Late reactions to food are more difficult to detect. Only a few studies have addressed this type of reaction, showing that about 25% of these reactions appear after 2 hours.[78,79] In addition, more than 10% of the children who reacted to an OFC developed isolated eczematous reactions after 16 hours or later.[79]

A combination of early noneczematous reactions and delayed eczematous reactions was described in more than 40% of the children who reacted to OFC.[76] Late reactions can occur infrequently as isolated reactions or after a previous immediate-type reaction. Several patients experienced an episode of increased cutaneous pruritus and transient morbilliform rash 6 to 10 hours after the initial immediate reaction to a positive challenge.[21] These late symptoms were less prominent than the immediate symptoms but tended to last for several hours. This type of reaction is suggestive of the "late phase" of an IgE-mediated response.[21]

The Diagnosis of Food Allergy in AD Patients

In the diagnosis of food allergy in AD patients, no single investigation is fully reliable alone and a stepwise approach, similar to those for other allergic disorders, is recommended in international guidelines for the diagnosis of food hypersensitivity.[76] The diagnostic workup of suspected food allergy should start with a detailed history and physical examination of the patient. The next step may include in vitro and/or in vivo allergy tests, that is, measurement of food-specific IgE antibodies, skin-prick tests, atopy patch tests (APT), diagnostic elimination diet, and/or oral challenge (**Fig. 2**).

The patient's history can be very helpful in identifying a potential relationship between symptoms and a specific food, especially for immediate, IgE-mediated reactions. In food-induced eczema, the predictive value of a positive case history is lower than that for food-induced immediate reactions. Parents and patients often attribute flares of eczema to the ingestion of certain foods. However, as a large number of other factors can lead to flares of eczema (*Staphylococcus* infection, irritants, heat and humidity, and so forth), the history is often not particularly informative, especially in patients with severe AD.[51,79,80] Sampson[21] showed that only 35% to 40% of parental reported suspicions of food allergy could be verified by DBPCFC.

When food allergy is suspected, in vivo tests (eg, skin-prick tests) and/or in vitro tests (eg, measurement of specific serum IgE) to assess IgE-mediated sensitization should be performed. Skin-prick tests done as first-line tests are useful for determining the presence of specific IgE antibodies to various foods. The list of tested foods should

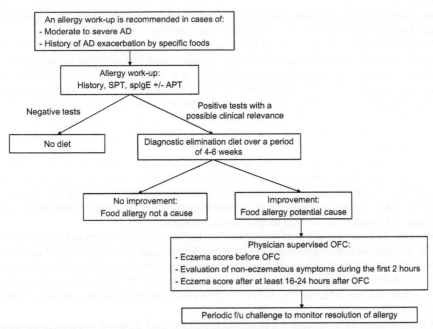

Fig. 2. Diagnostic algorithm for the identification of food allergy in AD. APT, atopy patch tests; f/u, follow-up; OFC, oral food challenge; SPT, skin-prick tests.

be adapted to the history and the age of the patient (**Table 4**). The negative predictive value of these tests is high (more than 95%), whereas the positive predictive value is low (approximately 40%).[56,57,81] This result suggests that a negative prick test can be helpful to rule out an allergy, but that a positive skin test cannot be considered to be diagnostic as such for a food allergy. Results need to be correlated with the clinical picture and, when necessary, confirmed by OFC.

Measurement of specific IgE antibodies in the blood by a standardized and validated method is also useful for detection of sensitization to food allergens, although

Table 4
Allergy testing in AD patients according to age

<3–4 Years	>3–4 Years
Foods (for AD-associated food allergy)	Foods (in case of severe persisting AD for AD-associated food allergy)
• Cow's milk	• Cow's milk
• Eggs	• Eggs
• (Peanuts, wheat, nuts, fish, and so forth)	• Peanuts
	• (Wheat, nuts, fish, and so forth)
Inhalant allergens (to test the atopic risk)	Inhalant allergens (for allergen-associated AD)
• House dust mites	• House dust mites
• Cat, dog, and other furred animals	• Cat, dog, and other furred animals
• Pollens	• Pollens

The allergen panel should be adjusted according to related symptomatology and local allergen exposure.
Data from Host A, Andrae S, Charkin S, et al. Allergy testing in children: why, who, when and how? Allergy 2003;58:559–69.

the sensitivity is lower. As with skin-prick tests, a negative result is helpful in excluding an IgE-mediated reaction to a specific food. A positive result has a lower specificity.[21] Quantitative measurements of food-specific IgE appear to be more useful in predicting clinical reactivity. Decision points have been established that provide greater than 95% confidence that a patient has symptomatic food allergy.[82,83] However, it has been well established that an OFC is needed to confirm food hypersensitivity when the level of specific IgE is lower than the cutoff point.

APT with common food allergens (milk, egg, wheat, and peanut) may increase the accuracy of food allergy diagnosis in patients with AD.[84–88] APT can be used as an additional diagnostic tool in specialized centers when skin-prick tests and/or specific IgE measurement fail to identify a suspected food or in patients with severe or persistent AD with a high suspicion of food allergy. APT can be also useful in patients with AD and multiple sensitizations without proven clinical relevance.[84] In these studies, children with immediate reactions generally had positive skin-prick tests whereas those with late reactions were more likely to have positive APT to the relevant foods. Studies using both skin-prick tests and APT to foods suggest that these tests are helpful in patients with delayed onset of symptoms.[84] However, APT still need to be standardized and are not yet recommended for routine clinical use.

Due to frequent skin flares and a high number of clinically nonrelevant positive tests in routine diagnostic procedures, the diagnosis of food allergy in AD patients can be difficult to establish based on skin or blood tests. Positive tests must be validated by a food elimination diet and most often by a controlled OFC.

Unfortunately, large numbers of patients with AD are started on empiric food elimination diets.[65] Although food allergens can be important triggers in AD, unnecessary elimination diets can cause malnutrition and significantly decrease the quality of life, in particular in children. Elimination diets should not be initiated based on a history-based suspicion alone. When a specific food is suspected by a positive allergy test, a diagnostic elimination diet over a period of up to 4 to 6 weeks with the suspected food items might be initiated.[76] If no food can be pinpointed by an allergy test in a patient with persistent moderate to severe AD, a diary reporting symptoms and food intake could be helpful in identifying a specific food.[21,71] If no association is found (note that this happens most of the time) and the diagnostic tests (prick tests, specific IgE ± APT) do not provide reliable information, an olligoallergenic diet over a period of 3 weeks can be helpful in patients with severe AD. In infants, an extensively hydrolyzed or amino acid formula can be used instead. Multiple dietary restrictions are rarely necessary and should be avoided.

Finally, standardized OFCs remain the "gold standard" for food allergy diagnosis in AD patients. If eczema remains stable or even increases in severity during a diagnostic elimination trial of 4 weeks, it is unlikely that the food is a relevant trigger of AD and an OFC is not necessary. If there is an improvement of the symptoms during a diagnostic elimination diet, an OFC should be performed, as the skin improvement may be coincidental or reflect a "placebo" effect, particularly in adults.[21,76] For patients with AD and prove noneczematous, immediate IgE-type reactions to a food will not need an OFC. In the investigation of active AD, a DBPCFC is highly recommended.[89] The OFC should always be performed by well-trained physicians and health personnel, and emergency equipment must be available (**Fig. 3**). Even when immediate reactions are not expected, the food must be administered with increasing doses as it may cause immediate, potentially severe symptoms, in particular in patients with AD on a long-lasting elimination of the incriminated food.[21] An OFC should only be performed in patients with stable skin condition. The extent of skin lesions should be scored, for example, by SCORAD (SCORing Atopic Dermatitis), before OFC and at least 24 hours

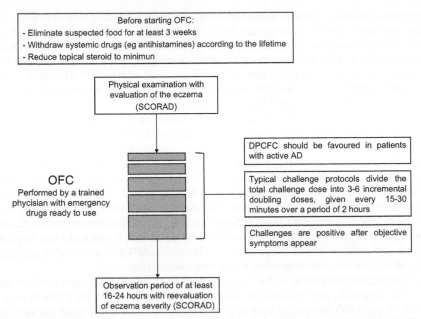

Fig. 3. Standard protocol for food challenges in patients with atopic dermatitis. OFC, oral food challenge; DPCFC, double-blind placebo-controlled food challenge.

later, as eczema flares related to the food might otherwise be overlooked. A difference of at least 10 SCORAD points is usually considered a positive reaction.[76] Other diagnostic tests, including the lymphocyte cytotoxicity test, basophil degranulation test, or measurement of food-specific IgG, are not validated and should not be used because they most often indicate a nonspecific immune reaction to the food and could be misleading.

Treatment of Food Allergy in AD Patients

In addition to management of AD with emollients, topical anti-inflammatory medications, antibiotics, and avoidance of environmental triggers, the only currently available treatment for patients with AD and food allergy is a strict dietary restriction of the causative food. As discussed earlier, long-term dietary avoidance should only be prescribed to patients with a well-documented diagnosis of food hypersensitivity. The avoidance diet needs to be thorough and carefully defined. The family and the patient must be taught how to read food labels to avoid potential sources of allergen contamination. In addition, patients and/or their parents need to be instructed to treat a potential reaction after accidental ingestion, and need to be equipped with an emergency treatment kit for anaphylaxis (antihistamines and self-injectable epinephrine) if there is a risk for systemic reaction. To date, treatment of food allergy by food-specific immunotherapy has not yet been proven to be safe and effective in well-designed trials, although oral desensitization trials are currently ongoing.

Follow-Up and Prognosis

AD starting in early infancy is often the first step of later manifestations of respiratory allergy known as the atopic march (see also the article by Jonathan M. Spergel elsewhere in this issue for further exploration of this topic). Food allergy is often associated with AD in patients presenting with this allergic phenotype. Approximately one-third of children with AD have a favorable outcome and will outgrow their food hypersensitivity over 1 to 3 years, depending on the food they are allergic to.[42] Allergy to egg white, cow's milk, or wheat is short lasting in most patients, whereas allergy to peanuts, nuts, fish, and shellfish may be long lasting. Children with AD-associated food allergy should be regularly reevaluated for persistence of allergy, for example, at intervals of 12 to 18 months, for milk or egg allergy. Peanut and tree nut allergies are most often long lasting and may need less frequent reevaluations. Measuring the level of serum-specific IgE for follow-up can be very helpful. Patients with an initial low level of specific IgE are more likely to outgrow their allergy than patients with a higher level. Following the positivity of skin-prick tests is not helpful, as they can remain positive for several years after the child has outgrown his food allergy. It has been suggested that patients who do not strictly avoid the offending food are less likely to lose their allergy.[21] To date, "no patients have experienced a recurrence of allergic symptoms or worsening of eczema once food hypersensitivity was lost."[21]

AD AND AEROALLERGENS

After the age of 3 years, the prevalence of food allergy decreases; however, sensitization to inhalant allergens becomes more common. It has been observed that patients with moderate or severe AD more often have positive IgE tests to house dust mites (HDM), molds, and fungi (eg, *Alternaria*) and yeasts (eg, *Malassezia*) than asthmatics or nonatopic controls.[48] The exact role of these sensitizations in the pathogenesis of AD remains controversial. However, in some patients contact with certain aeroallergens, such pollen or HDM, may trigger eczematous skin lesions.

Evidence Supporting the Role of Aeroallergens as AD Triggers

The role of aeroallergens in AD has not been investigated as extensively as food allergens. In 1918, Walker[90] observed that some of his AD patients had skin flares after contact with aeroallergens (horse, ragweed, timothy). Subsequently, Tuft found that most adult patients with AD displayed positive skin tests to HDM. He demonstrated that intranasal application of aeroallergens could exacerbate AD and that environmental avoidance of HDM would improve skin symptoms.[91,92] Later, Tupker and colleagues[93] reported that bronchoprovocation with a standardized HDM extract in a double-blind, randomized, placebo-controlled way can result in new-onset AD skin lesions and exacerbation of previously existing skin lesions. Together, these studies suggest that the respiratory route could be important in the induction and exacerbation of AD by aeroallergens.

Patch testing has been most extensively studied for inhalant allergens in AD. Epicutaneous application of aeroallergens on uninvolved skin of patients with AD by APT elicits eczematous reactions in a subset of patients.[48,94–98] Positive reactions have been observed to HDM, pollens, animal dander, and molds. In contrast, patients with respiratory allergy and healthy volunteers rarely have positive APT.[99] Positive APTs support a role for contact hypersensitivity to aeroallergens in AD. There are no definitive data to support either a primary role for aeroallergen sensitization through direct skin contact or indirectly by inhalation.[99]

At a cellular level, evidence supporting a role for aeroallergens in AD includes the presence of both allergen-specific IgE antibodies and allergen-specific T cells in the skin.[100] A recent study found that 95% of AD patients were positive for IgE to HDM as compared with 42% of asthmatic patients.[48] Moreover, the HDM-specific IgE titers were usually at least 20-fold higher in AD than in asthma patients. Evidence of HDM (and other aeroallergen)–specific T cells in lesional skin and at the site of positive

HDM patch test supports the concept that immune responses in AD skin can be elicited by percutaneous exposure to aeroallergens.[25] Using the APT, Langeveld-Wildschut and colleagues[101] showed that positive reactions to HDM were associated with IgE-positive LC in the epidermis of AD patients. Together, these studies support, at the clinical and cellular levels, the importance of aeroallergens in a subgroup of patients with AD.

Common Aeroallergens Incriminated in AD

As discussed above, aeroallergens can exacerbate AD either by inhalation or by direct contact with the skin. Relevant allergens include HDM (most frequently incriminated), animal dander, and pollen. Fungus and cockroach have been suspected as well.[102,103] However, well-controlled clinical studies have validated only HDM as a clear trigger for AD.

Diagnosis of Aeroallergen Allergy in AD Patients

Similarly to food allergy, the diagnosis is based on a sequential allergy workup. History can be particularly helpful to identify pollens (seasonal flares) or animal dander allergens as triggers of AD. In a second step, skin-prick tests or measurements of specific IgE antibodies are useful to detect sensitization to aeroallergens. Allergens should be selected according to the history and the age of the patients (see **Table 4**). Similarly to foods, the severity of AD has been correlated with the degree of sensitization to aeroallergens.[104]

In addition to skin-prick tests and specific IgE, APT can be used to assess a skin-specific response to various aeroallergens, including HDM, pollen, animal dander, and molds. Patch testing elicits eczematous reactions in 15% to 100% of patients with AD, according to patch test materials and test modalities.[94–98] Based on the history of aeroallergen-triggered AD flares, APT has proved to have a higher specificity but lower sensitivity than skin-prick tests or specific IgE.[105] In 2003, Kerschenlohr and colleagues[106] reported positive APT in patients with nonatopic eczema,[106] suggesting that aeroallergens might also be relevant triggers for nonatopic eczema, even in the absence of detectable aeroallergen-specific serum IgE and with negative skin-prick test (SPT) results.

Recently, the European Academy of Allergy and Clinical Immunology (EAACI) suggested the following indications for APT[84]:

- Suspicion of aeroallergen-related symptoms in absence of positive specific IgE and/or a positive SPT
- Severe and/or persistent AD with unknown triggering factors
- Multiple IgE sensitizations without proven clinical relevance in patients with AD.

APT might become an important diagnostic tool, especially in patients with nonatopic eczema in whom SPTs and serum IgE tests fail to identify relevant allergens. The major problem with APT is the variability of methods and results among investigators.[107,108] Thus, standardization of the procedure is needed. Although hampered by the absence of a gold standard for aeroallergen-induced eczema diagnosis, specific avoidance measures should be considered in patients with positive APT.

Treatment of Aeroallergen Allergy in AD Patients

Several studies have examined whether avoidance of aeroallergens may improve AD. Most of these studies have focused on HDM allergy and have shown a positive effect of HDM avoidance measures.[105] These reports are mostly uncontrolled trials in which patients were in dust mite–free environments, such as hospital rooms, or by use of acaricides or dust mite–proof encasing. All these measures have led to improvement of AD.[99] A double-blind, placebo-controlled study using a combination of effective mite reduction measures in the home showed that lower levels of HDM are associated with significant improvement of AD.[109] By contrast, other studies have found no clinical benefit from HDM avoidance,[110,111] even though encasing resulted in a significant decrease in HDM allergen levels.

In addition to avoidance, specific immunotherapy (SIT) could be an effective therapeutic intervention. A potential role of SIT in environmental allergen-triggered AD has been shown in several case reports and smaller cohort studies,[112] as well as recently in a multicenter trial with HDM immunotherapy involving 51 patients.[113] As a result of these studies, it became clear that SIT used for treatment of patients with allergic rhinitis and/or asthma can also be used in patients with AD, as eczema was not worsened during or after SIT. This finding suggests a potential benefit of SIT for AD in patients primarily treated for allergic rhinitis or mild asthma. However, even if there are several studies showing a positive effect of SIT on AD, no definite conclusion on the efficiency of SIT in AD can be drawn at present.[112] Prospective studies involving larger numbers of patients are currently being performed, which may answer the question of whether AD alone could be an indication for the initiation of SIT.

DIRECT ALLERGEN SKIN CONTACT

AD patients were previously thought to be less prone to develop contact allergy, although it is known today that the prevalence of delayed-type sensitization to common allergens (fragrances, latex and rubber accelerators, lanolin, and formaldehyde) in AD patients is as frequent as in nonatopic individuals[114,115] (see the article by Fonacier and Aquino elsewhere in this issue for further exploration of this topic). Therefore, preventive measures should begin early in life to avoid contact with common sensitizers. Contact dermatitis should always be considered as a potential flare-up trigger in AD. Patch tests to common allergens (including topical medications), cosmetic products (emollients), and even corticosteroids should be performed when suspected in AD patients.

SUMMARY

After years of debate and uncertainties, it is now clear that allergens may play a significant pathogenic role in a subgroup of patients with AD and can be considered as specific triggers of AD. Therapeutic measures, such as elimination of the incriminated allergen(s), can lead to marked improvement of AD; this is particularly true for food allergens but also for inhalant allergens. Patient care should include early allergy diagnosis by SPTs, specific IgE test and/or APT, and when necessary, OFC.

REFERENCES

1. Johansson SG, Bieber T, Dahl R, et al. Revised nomenclature for allergy for global use: Report of the Nomenclature Review Committee of the World Allergy Organization, October 2003. J Allergy Clin Immunol 2004;113(5):832–6.
2. Worldwide variation in prevalence of symptoms of asthma, allergic rhinoconjunctivitis, and atopic eczema: ISAAC. The International Study of Asthma and Allergies in Childhood (ISAAC) Steering Committee. Lancet 1998;351(9111):1225–32.
3. Kay J, Gawkrodger DJ, Mortimer MJ, et al. The prevalence of childhood atopic eczema in a general population. J Am Acad Dermatol 1994;30(1):35–9.

4. Cabon N, Ducombs G, Mortureux P, et al. Contact allergy to aeroallergens in children with atopic dermatitis: comparison with allergic contact dermatitis. Contact Dermatitis 1996;35(1):27–32.

5. Bohme M, Wickman M, Lennart Nordvall S, et al. Family history and risk of atopic dermatitis in children up to 4 years. Clin Exp Allergy 2003;33(9):1226–31.

6. Schmid-Grendelmeier P, Simon D, Simon HU, et al. Epidemiology, clinical features, and immunology of the "intrinsic" (non-IgE-mediated) type of atopic dermatitis (constitutional dermatitis). Allergy 2001;56(9):841–9.

7. Akdis CA, Akdis M, Bieber T, et al. Diagnosis and treatment of atopic dermatitis in children and adults: European Academy of Allergology and Clinical Immunology/American Academy of Allergy, Asthma and Immunology/PRACTALL Consensus Report. J Allergy Clin Immunol 2006;118(1):152–69.

8. Cork MJ, Robinson DA, Vasilopoulos Y, et al. New perspectives on epidermal barrier dysfunction in atopic dermatitis: gene-environment interactions. J Allergy Clin Immunol 2006;118(1):3–21 [quiz: 22–3].

9. Adinoff AD, Tellez P, Clark RA. Atopic dermatitis and aeroallergen contact sensitivity. J Allergy Clin Immunol 1988;81(4):736–42.

10. Lack G, Fox D, Northstone K, et al. Factors associated with the development of peanut allergy in childhood. N Engl J Med 2003;348(11):977–85.

11. Brunner M, Walzer M. Absorption of undigested proteins in human beings: the absorption of unaltered fish protein in adults. Arch Intern Med 1928;42:173–9.

12. Walzer M. Absorption of allergens. J Allergy 1942;13:554–62.

13. Berin MC, Kiliaan AJ, Yang PC, et al. Rapid transepithelial antigen transport in rat jejunum: impact of sensitization and the hypersensitivity reaction. Gastroenterology 1997;113(3):856–64.

14. Berin MC, Kiliaan AJ, Yang PC, et al. The influence of mast cells on pathways of transepithelial antigen transport in rat intestine. J Immunol 1998;161(5):2561–6.

15. Prescott VE, Forbes E, Foster PS, et al. Mechanistic analysis of experimental food allergen-induced cutaneous reactions. J Leukoc Biol 2006;80(2):258–66.

16. Sampson HA. Food sensitivity and the pathogenesis of atopic dermatitis. J R Soc Med 1997;90(Suppl 30):2–8.

17. Novak N, Bieber T, Leung DY. Immune mechanisms leading to atopic dermatitis. J Allergy Clin Immunol 2003;112(6 Suppl):S128–39.

18. Spiegelberg HL. Structure and function of Fc receptors for IgE on lymphocytes, monocytes, and macrophages. Adv Immunol 1984;35:61–88.

19. Joseph M, Capron A, Ameisen JC, et al. The receptor for IgE on blood platelets. Eur J Immunol 1986;16(3):306–12.

20. Capron M, Capron A, Joseph M, et al. IgE receptors on phagocytic cells and immune response to schistosome infection. Monogr Allergy 1983;18:33–44.

21. Sampson HA. The evaluation and management of food allergy in atopic dermatitis. Clin Dermatol 2003;21(3):183–92.

22. Baud O, Goulet O, Canioni D, et al. Treatment of the immune dysregulation, polyendocrinopathy, enteropathy, X-linked syndrome (IPEX) by allogeneic bone marrow transplantation. N Engl J Med 2001;344(23):1758–62.

23. Spergel JM, Mizoguchi E, Oettgen H, et al. Roles of TH1 and TH2 cytokines in a murine model of allergic dermatitis. J Clin Invest 1999;103(8):1103–11.

24. van Reijsen FC, Felius A, Wauters EA, et al. T-cell reactivity for a peanut-derived epitope in the skin of a young infant with atopic dermatitis. J Allergy Clin Immunol 1998;101(2 Pt 1):207–9.

25. van Reijsen FC, Bruijnzeel-Koomen CA, Kalthoff FS, et al. Skin-derived aeroallergen-specific T-cell clones of Th2 phenotype in patients with atopic dermatitis. J Allergy Clin Immunol 1992;90(2):184–93.
26. Reekers R, Beyer K, Niggemann B, et al. The role of circulating food antigen-specific lymphocytes in food allergic children with atopic dermatitis. Br J Dermatol 1996;135(6):935–41.
27. Werfel T, Ahlers G, Schmidt P, et al. Detection of a kappa-casein-specific lymphocyte response in milk-responsive atopic dermatitis. Clin Exp Allergy 1996;26(12):1380–6.
28. Abernathy-Carver KJ, Sampson HA, Picker LJ, et al. Milk-induced eczema is associated with the expansion of T cells expressing cutaneous lymphocyte antigen. J Clin Invest 1995;95(2):913–8.
29. Beyer K, Castro R, Feidel C, et al. Milk-induced urticaria is associated with the expansion of T cells expressing cutaneous lymphocyte antigen. J Allergy Clin Immunol 2002;109(4):688–93.
30. Wakita H, Sakamoto T, Tokura Y, et al. E-selectin and vascular cell adhesion molecule-1 as critical adhesion molecules for infiltration of T lymphocytes and eosinophils in atopic dermatitis. J Cutan Pathol 1994;21(1):33–9.
31. Schon MP, Zollner TM, Boehncke WH. The molecular basis of lymphocyte recruitment to the skin: clues for pathogenesis and selective therapies of inflammatory disorders. J Invest Dermatol 2003;121(5):951–62.
32. Kallos P, Kallos L. Experimental asthma in guinea pigs revisited. Int Arch Allergy Appl Immunol 1984;73(1):77–85.
33. Lin W, Truong N, Grossman WJ, et al. Allergic dysregulation and hyperimmunoglobulinemia E in Foxp3 mutant mice. J Allergy Clin Immunol 2005;116(5):1106–15.
34. Kiehl P, Falkenberg K, Vogelbruch M, et al. Tissue eosinophilia in acute and chronic atopic dermatitis: a morphometric approach using quantitative image analysis of immunostaining. Br J Dermatol 2001;145(5):720–9.
35. Pucci N, Lombardi E, Novembre E, et al. Urinary eosinophil protein X and serum eosinophil cationic protein in infants and young children with atopic dermatitis: correlation with disease activity. J Allergy Clin Immunol 2000; 105(2 Pt 1):353–7.
36. Leiferman KM, Ackerman SJ, Sampson HA, et al. Dermal deposition of eosinophil-granule major basic protein in atopic dermatitis. Comparison with onchocerciasis. N Engl J Med 1985;313(5):282–5.
37. Sampson HA, Jolie PL. Increased plasma histamine concentrations after food challenges in children with atopic dermatitis. N Engl J Med 1984;311(6):372–6.
38. Suomalainen H, Soppi E, Isolauri E. Evidence for eosinophil activation in cow's milk allergy. Pediatr Allergy Immunol 1994;5(1):27–31.
39. Niggemann B, Beyer K, Wahn U. The role of eosinophils and eosinophil cationic protein in monitoring oral challenge tests in children with food-sensitive atopic dermatitis. J Allergy Clin Immunol 1994;94(6 Pt 1):963–71.
40. Schnyder B, Lugli S, Feng N, et al. Interleukin-4 (IL-4) and IL-13 bind to a shared heterodimeric complex on endothelial cells mediating vascular cell adhesion molecule-1 induction in the absence of the common gamma chain. Blood 1996;87(10):4286–95.
41. Hamid Q, Boguniewicz M, Leung DY. Differential in situ cytokine gene expression in acute versus chronic atopic dermatitis. J Clin Invest 1994;94(2):870–6.
42. Sampson HA, Broadbent KR, Bernhisel-Broadbent J. Spontaneous release of histamine from basophils and histamine-releasing factor in patients with atopic dermatitis and food hypersensitivity. N Engl J Med 1989;321(4):228–32.

43. Sampson HA, MacDonald SM. IgE-dependent histamine-releasing factors. Springer Semin Immunopathol 1993;15(1):89–98.
44. Lyczak JB, Zhang K, Saxon A, et al. Expression of novel secreted isoforms of human immunoglobulin E proteins. J Biol Chem 1996;271(7):3428–36.
45. Leung DY. Infection in atopic dermatitis. Curr Opin Pediatr 2003;15(4):399–404.
46. Leung DY, Harbeck R, Bina P, et al. Presence of IgE antibodies to staphylococcal exotoxins on the skin of patients with atopic dermatitis. Evidence for a new group of allergens. J Clin Invest 1993;92(3):1374–80.
47. Bunikowski R, Mielke M, Skarabis H, et al. Prevalence and role of serum IgE antibodies to the *Staphylococcus aureus*-derived superantigens SEA and SEB in children with atopic dermatitis. J Allergy Clin Immunol 1999;103(1 Pt 1):119–24.
48. Scalabrin DM, Bavbek S, Perzanowski MS, et al. Use of specific IgE in assessing the relevance of fungal and dust mite allergens to atopic dermatitis: a comparison with asthmatic and nonasthmatic control subjects. J Allergy Clin Immunol 1999;104(6):1273–9.
49. Mothes N, Niggemann B, Jenneck C, et al. The cradle of IgE autoreactivity in atopic eczema lies in early infancy. J Allergy Clin Immunol 2005;116(3):706–9.
50. Schloss OM. Allergy to common foods. Trans Am Pediatr Soc 1915;27:62–8.
51. Atherton DJ, Sewell M, Soothill JF, et al. A double-blind controlled crossover trial of an antigen-avoidance diet in atopic eczema. Lancet 1978;1(8061):401–3.
52. Juto P, Engberg S, Winberg J. Treatment of infantile atopic dermatitis with a strict elimination diet. Clin Allergy 1978;8(5):493–500.
53. Hill DJ, Lynch BC. Elemental diet in the management of severe eczema in childhood. Clin Allergy 1982;12(3):313–5.
54. Neild VS, Marsden RA, Bailes JA, et al. Egg and milk exclusion diets in atopic eczema. Br J Dermatol 1986;114(1):117–23.
55. Lever R, MacDonald C, Waugh P, et al. Randomised controlled trial of advice on an egg exclusion diet in young children with atopic eczema and sensitivity to eggs. Pediatr Allergy Immunol 1998;9(1):13–9.
56. Bock SA, Lee WY, Remigio L, et al. Appraisal of skin tests with food extracts for diagnosis of food hypersensitivity. Clin Allergy 1978;8(6):559–64.
57. Sampson HA. Role of immediate food hypersensitivity in the pathogenesis of atopic dermatitis. J Allergy Clin Immunol 1983;71(5):473–80.
58. Sampson HA, McCaskill CC. Food hypersensitivity and atopic dermatitis: evaluation of 113 patients. J Pediatr 1985;107(5):669–75.
59. Sampson HA. Atopic dermatitis. Ann Allergy 1992;69(6):469–79.
60. Kramer MS, Kakuma R. Maternal dietary antigen avoidance during pregnancy and/or lactation for preventing or treating atopic disease in the child. Cochrane Database Syst Rev 2003;4:CD000133.
61. Fergusson DM, Horwood LJ, Shannon FT. Early solid feeding and recurrent childhood eczema: a 10-year longitudinal study. Pediatrics 1990;86(4):541–6.
62. Kajosaari M. Atopy prophylaxis in high-risk infants. Prospective 5-year follow-up study of children with six months exclusive breastfeeding and solid food elimination. Adv Exp Med Biol 1991;310:453–8.
63. Osterballe M, Hansen TK, Mortz CG, et al. The prevalence of food hypersensitivity in an unselected population of children and adults. Pediatr Allergy Immunol 2005;16(7):567–73.
64. Guillet G, Guillet MH. Natural history of sensitizations in atopic dermatitis. A 3-year follow-up in 250 children: food allergy and high risk of respiratory symptoms. Arch Dermatol 1992;128(2):187–92.

65. Sicherer SH, Sampson HA. Food hypersensitivity and atopic dermatitis: patho-physiology, epidemiology, diagnosis, and management. J Allergy Clin Immunol 1999;104(3 Pt 2):S114–22.
66. Eigenmann PA, Calza AM. Diagnosis of IgE-mediated food allergy among Swiss children with atopic dermatitis. Pediatr Allergy Immunol 2000;11(2):95–100.
67. Munkvad M, Danielsen L, Hoj L, et al. Antigen-free diet in adult patients with atopic dermatitis. A double-blind controlled study. Acta Derm Venereol 1984; 64(6):524–8.
68. de Maat-Bleeker F, Bruijnzeel-Koomen C. Food allergy in adults with atopic dermatitis. Monogr Allergy 1996;32:157–63.
69. Woods RK, Thien F, Raven J, et al. Prevalence of food allergies in young adults and their relationship to asthma, nasal allergies, and eczema. Ann Allergy Asthma Immunol 2002;88(2):183–9.
70. Uenishi T, Sugiura H, Uehara M. Role of foods in irregular aggravation of atopic dermatitis. J Dermatol 2003;30(2):91–7.
71. Werfel T, Erdmann S, Fuchs T, et al. Approach to suspected food allergy in atopic dermatitis. Guideline of the Task Force on Food Allergy of the German Society of Allergology and Clinical Immunology (DGAKI) and the Medical Association of German Allergologists (ADA) and the German Society of Pediatric Allergology (GPA). J Dtsch Dermatol Ges 2009;7(3):265–71.
72. Worm M, Ehlers I, Sterry W, et al. Clinical relevance of food additives in adult patients with atopic dermatitis. Clin Exp Allergy 2000;30(3):407–14.
73. Ehlers I, Worm M, Sterry W, et al. Sugar is not an aggravating factor in atopic dermatitis. Acta Derm Venereol 2001;81(4):282–4.
74. Breuer K, Wulf A, Constien A, et al. Birch pollen-related food as a provocation factor of allergic symptoms in children with atopic eczema/dermatitis syndrome. Allergy 2004;59(9):988–94.
75. Worm M, Forschner K, Lee HH, et al. Frequency of atopic dermatitis and relevance of food allergy in adults in Germany. Acta Derm Venereol 2006;86(2):119–22.
76. Werfel T, Ballmer-Weber B, Eigenmann PA, et al. Eczematous reactions to food in atopic eczema: position paper of the EAACI and GA2LEN. Allergy 2007;62(7): 723–8.
77. Strobel S, Ferguson A. Immune responses to fed protein antigens in mice. 3. Systemic tolerance or priming is related to age at which antigen is first encountered. Pediatr Res 1984;18(7):588–94.
78. Celik-Bilgili S, Mehl A, Verstege A, et al. The predictive value of specific immunoglobulin E levels in serum for the outcome of oral food challenges. Clin Exp Allergy 2005;35(3):268–73.
79. Breuer K, Heratizadeh A, Wulf A, et al. Late eczematous reactions to food in children with atopic dermatitis. Clin Exp Allergy 2004;34(5):817–24.
80. Niggemann B, Sielaff B, Beyer K, et al. Outcome of double-blind, placebo-controlled food challenge tests in 107 children with atopic dermatitis. Clin Exp Allergy 1999;29(1):91–6.
81. Sampson HA, Albergo R. Comparison of results of skin tests, RAST, and double-blind, placebo-controlled food challenges in children with atopic dermatitis. J Allergy Clin Immunol 1984;74(1):26–33.
82. Sampson HA, Ho DG. Relationship between food-specific IgE concentrations and the risk of positive food challenges in children and adolescents. J Allergy Clin Immunol 1997;100(4):444–51.
83. Sampson HA. Utility of food-specific IgE concentrations in predicting symptomatic food allergy. J Allergy Clin Immunol 2001;107(5):891–6.

84. Turjanmaa K, Darsow U, Niggemann B, et al. EAACI/GA2LEN position paper: present status of the atopy patch test. Allergy 2006;61(12):1377–84.
85. Kekki OM, Turjanmaa K, Isolauri E. Differences in skin-prick and patch-test reactivity are related to the heterogeneity of atopic eczema in infants. Allergy 1997; 52(7):755–9.
86. Majamaa H, Moisio P, Holm K, et al. Cow's milk allergy: diagnostic accuracy of skin prick and patch tests and specific IgE. Allergy 1999;54(4):346–51.
87. Niggemann B, Reibel S, Wahn U. The atopy patch test (APT)—a useful tool for the diagnosis of food allergy in children with atopic dermatitis. Allergy 2000; 55(3):281–5.
88. Saarinen KM, Suomalainen H, Savilahti E. Diagnostic value of skin-prick and patch tests and serum eosinophil cationic protein and cow's milk-specific IgE in infants with cow's milk allergy. Clin Exp Allergy 2001;31(3):423–9.
89. Niggemann B. Role of oral food challenges in the diagnostic work-up of food allergy in atopic eczema dermatitis syndrome. Allergy 2004;59(Suppl 78):32–4.
90. Walker I. Causation of eczema, urticaria and angioneurotic edema. J Am Med Assoc 1918;70:897.
91. Tuft L. Importance of inhalant allergens in atopic dermatitis. J Invest Dermatol 1949;12(4):211–9.
92. Tuft L, Heck VM. Studies in atopic dermatitis. IV. Importance of seasonal inhalant allergens, especially ragweed. J Allergy 1952;23(6):528–40.
93. Tupker RA, De Monchy JG, Coenraads PJ, et al. Induction of atopic dermatitis by inhalation of house dust mite. J Allergy Clin Immunol 1996;97(5):1064–70.
94. Ring J, Darsow U, Gfesser M, et al. The 'atopy patch test' in evaluating the role of aeroallergens in atopic eczema. Int Arch Allergy Immunol 1997;113(1–3):379–83.
95. Seidenari S, Manzini BM, Danese P. Patch testing with pollens of Gramineae in patients with atopic dermatitis and mucosal atopy. Contact Dermatitis 1992; 27(2):125–6.
96. Darsow U, Vieluf D, Ring J. Atopy patch test with different vehicles and allergen concentrations: an approach to standardization. J Allergy Clin Immunol 1995; 95(3):677–84.
97. Seidenari S, Giusti F, Pellacani G, et al. Frequency and intensity of responses to mite patch tests are lower in nonatopic subjects with respect to patients with atopic dermatitis. Allergy 2003;58(5):426–9.
98. Darsow U, Laifaoui J, Kerschenlohr K, et al. The prevalence of positive reactions in the atopy patch test with aeroallergens and food allergens in subjects with atopic eczema: a European multicenter study. Allergy 2004;59(12):1318–25.
99. Dai YS. Allergens in atopic dermatitis. Clin Rev Allergy Immunol 2007;33(3): 157–66.
100. van der Heijden FL, Wierenga EA, Bos JD, et al. High frequency of IL-4-producing CD4+ allergen-specific T lymphocytes in atopic dermatitis lesional skin. J Invest Dermatol 1991;97(3):389–94.
101. Langeveld-Wildschut EG, Bruijnzeel PL, Mudde GC, et al. Clinical and immunologic variables in skin of patients with atopic eczema and either positive or negative atopy patch test reactions. J Allergy Clin Immunol 2000;105(5): 1008–16.
102. Simon-Nobbe B, Denk U, Poll V, et al. The spectrum of fungal allergy. Int Arch Allergy Immunol 2008;145(1):58–86.
103. Michel S, Yawalkar N, Schnyder B, et al. Eczematous skin reaction to atopy patch testing with cockroach in patients with atopic dermatitis. J Investig Allergol Clin Immunol 2009;19(3):173–9.

104. Darsow U, Ring J. Airborne and dietary allergens in atopic eczema: a comprehensive review of diagnostic tests. Clin Exp Dermatol 2000;25(7):544–51.
105. Darsow U, Wollenberg A, Simon D, et al. ETFAD/EADV eczema task force 2009 position paper on diagnosis and treatment of atopic dermatitis. J Eur Acad Dermatol Venereol 2010;24(3):317–28.
106. Kerschenlohr K, Decard S, Przybilla B, et al. Atopy patch test reactions show a rapid influx of inflammatory dendritic epidermal cells in patients with extrinsic atopic dermatitis and patients with intrinsic atopic dermatitis. J Allergy Clin Immunol 2003;111(4):869–74.
107. Heinemann C, Schliemann-Willers S, Kelterer D, et al. The atopy patch test—reproducibility and comparison of different evaluation methods. Allergy 2002; 57(7):641–5.
108. Bygum A, Mortz CG, Andersen KE. Atopy patch tests in young adult patients with atopic dermatitis and controls: dose-response relationship, objective reading, reproducibility and clinical interpretation. Acta Derm Venereol 2003; 83(1):18–23.
109. Tan BB, Weald D, Strickland I, et al. Double-blind controlled trial of effect of housedust-mite allergen avoidance on atopic dermatitis. Lancet 1996; 347(8993):15–8.
110. Oosting AJ, de Bruin-Weller MS, Terreehorst I, et al. Effect of mattress encasings on atopic dermatitis outcome measures in a double-blind, placebo-controlled study: the Dutch mite avoidance study. J Allergy Clin Immunol 2002;110(3): 500–6.
111. Koopman LP, van Strien RT, Kerkhof M, et al. Placebo-controlled trial of house dust mite-impermeable mattress covers: effect on symptoms in early childhood. Am J Respir Crit Care Med 2002;166(3):307–13.
112. Bussmann C, Bockenhoff A, Henke H, et al. Does allergen-specific immunotherapy represent a therapeutic option for patients with atopic dermatitis? J Allergy Clin Immunol 2006;118(6):1292–8.
113. Werfel T, Breuer K, Rueff F, et al. Usefulness of specific immunotherapy in patients with atopic dermatitis and allergic sensitization to house dust mites: a multi-centre, randomized, dose-response study. Allergy 2006;61(2):202–5.
114. Lever R, Forsyth A. Allergic contact dermatitis in atopic dermatitis. Acta Derm Venereol Suppl (Stockh) 1992;176:95–8.
115. Marks JG Jr, Belsito DV, DeLeo VA, et al. North American Contact Dermatitis Group patch-test results, 1996–1998. Arch Dermatol 2000;136(2):272–3.

The Infectious Aspects of Atopic Dermatitis

Peck Y. Ong, MD[a,b], Donald Y.M. Leung, MD, PhD[c,d],*

KEYWORDS

- *S aureus* - Eczema herpeticum - Eczema vaccinatum
- Superantigen - Toll-like receptors - Malassezia

Atopic dermatitis (AD) is a chronic inflammatory skin disease that causes significant morbidity in affected individuals. The disease is often characterized by chronic inflammation and pruritus interrupted by acute flares and bacterial infection.[1] AD results in significant sleep loss, poor school/work performance, and disruption of social activities. In addition, severe AD patients are at risk for rare invasive bacterial infections and life-threatening eczema herpeticum (EH).[2,3] Although recent studies have provided strong support for the basis of skin barrier defects in the pathogenesis of AD,[4] the cause of AD remains incompletely understood. More recent data have also provided further insights into the important role of immune responses in the pathogenesis of AD (**Table 1**). Of note, AD patients with increased allergic responses have more severe skin disease and a greater tendency to suffer from skin infections. These studies provide evidence for a role of the immune response in the expression of AD. Secondary skin infections have long been known to be associated with AD flare. The most common skin infections in AD are caused by *Staphylococcus aureus* and herpes simplex virus (HSV). In the absence of clinical signs of infections, most AD patients are also colonized with *S aureus* on their skin lesions. This pathogen is known to produce a myriad of proinflammatory factors that may trigger the cutaneous immune system.[5] In this review, the authors discuss

[a] Division of Clinical Immunology and Allergy, Childrens Hospital Los Angeles, 4650 Sunset Boulevard, MS #75, Los Angeles, CA 90027, USA
[b] Department of Pediatrics, Keck School of Medicine, University of Southern California, Los Angeles, CA, USA
[c] Division of Pediatric Allergy-Immunology, National Jewish Health, 1400 Jackson Street, Denver, CO 80206, USA
[d] Department of Pediatrics, University of Colorado Denver, Denver, CO, USA
* Corresponding author. Division of Pediatric Allergy-Immunology, National Jewish Health, 1400 Jackson Street, Denver, CO 80206.
E-mail address: leungd@njhealth.org

Immunol Allergy Clin N Am 30 (2010) 309–321
doi:10.1016/j.iac.2010.05.001
0889-8561/10/$ – see front matter © 2010 Elsevier Inc. All rights reserved.

immunology.theclinics.com

Table 1
Recent developments in the infectious aspects of AD
Filaggrin gene mutations facilitate IgE expression in a mouse model[20]
Toll-like receptor genetic polymorphisms may lead to cytokine dysregulation and inflammation in AD[45–47]
Emerging roles of nonclassical staphylococcal superantigens (SEE and SEG-SEQ) and methicillin-resistant *Staphylococcus aureus* in the pathogenesis of AD[5,58,59]
AD patients with specific IgE sensitization or other atopic diseases including asthma and food allergy are at increased risk for viral skin infections[67]
Innate immune response genes including leukotriene B4 receptor (LTB4R), orosomucoid 1 (ORM1), coagulation factor II (thrombin) receptor (F2R), complement component 9 (C9), lipopolysaccharide binding protein (LBP), and leucine-rich repeat protein 1 (NLRP1) may be involved in the pathogenesis of vaccinia virus infection in AD[74]

recent developments in the genetic basis of skin barrier, immune phenotypes, and the role of microbial pathogens in AD.

SKIN BARRIER DEFECTS IN THE PATHOGENESIS OF AD

The stratum corneum (SC) of the skin acts as an important barrier in preventing water loss from the skin and in protecting the skin from intrusion by irritants or microbes. Based mainly on transepidermal water loss (TEWL) studies, the SC of AD skin has been found to be defective. The TEWL in AD lesions is significantly greater as compared with nonlesional AD skin and healthy skin.[6,7] In addition, it has been shown that nonlesional AD skin has greater TEWL and significantly thinner SC than healthy skin (12.2 μm vs 19.7 μm).[8] Increased TEWL correlates with increased AD severity.[9] Various proteins and lipids responsible for skin barrier function have been found to be deficient in AD skin. These molecules include filaggrin, involcrin, cholesterol, free fatty acids, and ceramides.[10,11] More recently, a genetic basis for the skin barrier defect in AD has been demonstrated by the strong association between filaggrin gene mutations and AD.[4] Two loss-of-function mutations in the filaggrin gene (FLG) (R501X and 2282del4) have been linked to childhood-onset AD, particularly in patients who have onset of AD at 2 years or younger.[12] Of patients with onset of AD 2 years or younger, 21.3% had 1 or more FLG mutated alleles, as compared with 15.8% and 9.5% in patients with non-FLG related childhood-onset AD and healthy controls, respectively.[12] These results were also replicated in AD patients with rarer FLG mutations such as R2447X, S3247X, 3702delG, and 3673delC.[13] In addition, it has been shown that patients with early-onset AD and FLG mutations have a tendency to have persistent disease into adulthood.[14] FLG in AD patients was significantly associated with the extrinsic form of the disease (ie, patients with elevated total serum IgE and/or presence of specific IgE against inhalant or food allergens), and the development of allergic rhinitis and asthma.[15–19] The association of IgE sensitization with FLG in AD has recently been supported by a mouse model with a homozygous frameshift mutation in filaggrin that is analogous to human FLG.[20] This mouse model facilitates cutaneous allergen sensitization that leads to production of specific IgE. Although the association of FLG with AD and atopy is clear, the role of FLG in modifying immune response in human AD has not been established. Of note, approximately 40% of carriers of FLG mutations showed no sign of AD.[4] Indeed, FLG mutations were initially found to be the cause of ichthyosis vulgaris, which is a dry skin condition with no apparent inflammation or infection.[21] Therefore, additional factors must be involved in the pathogenesis of AD.

SUSCEPTIBILITY OF AD PATIENTS TO INFECTIONS

Psoriasis is another chronic skin disease with skin barrier defects. Based on TEWL experiments, psoriasis and AD were found to have a similar physical barrier dysfunction.[6] However, AD is associated with recurrent bacterial or viral infection, whereas secondary infection in psoriasis is uncommon.[22] A deficiency in host defense molecules may contribute to the increased infections in AD. Sphingosine, a skin lipid with anti–S aureus activity, has been shown to be significantly decreased in AD skin and lesions as compared with healthy skin.[23] A decrease in dermcidin, an antimicrobial peptide (AMP) produced by eccrine sweat glands, has also been found in AD.[24] Two major classes of AMPs in cutaneous innate immunity, β-defensins and a cathelicidin (LL-37), have also been shown to be decreased in AD as compared with psoriasis.[25,26] In addition to a deficiency in the first-line defense against microbial pathogens, adaptive immunity may also play a role in perpetuating susceptibility of AD to infections. Cell wall components of S aureus have been implicated as a trigger for the production of thymic stromal lymphopoietin (TSLP) by epithelial cells including keratinocytes.[27] This cytokine increases the production of T-helper 2 (Th2)-associated chemokines, CCL17 and CCL20, by macrophages or dendritic cells, leading to increased infiltration of Th2 cells, which express increased levels of Th2 cytokines, interleukin (IL-4) and IL-13. These cytokines favor the attachment of S aureus to AD skin.[28] IL-4 and IL-13 also suppress filaggrin expression, contributing to further barrier compromise in AD.[29] In addition, IL-4 and IL-13 also suppress AMP expression by keratinocytes.[25,26] These 2 cytokines were shown to suppress the expression of human β defensin-3, a key β-defensin against S aureus, via the inhibition of mobilization of this AMP in keratinocyte, rather than via the suppression of gene expression.[30] IL-17 is a T-cell cytokine that is capable of up-regulating the expression of AMPs in keratinocytes.[31] Decreased IL-17 expression in AD lesions, as compared with that in psoriasis, may contribute to the reduced AMP expression in AD.[32] Th2 cytokines may further suppress IL-17 expression in keratinocytes,[33] leading to lower expression of AMP in AD as compared with that in psoriasis.

Environmental factors may also play a role in the increased colonization of S aureus in AD. Patients with more severe AD have a higher level of S aureus found in their home environment.[34] A mechanism for recolonization of S aureus in AD patients from the environment has been supported by studies showing that AD patients and their close contacts have the same strains of S aureus based on molecular techniques.[35,36] In addition, topical medications that are contaminated with S aureus may become a source of bacterial recolonization in AD patients.[37]

THE ROLE OF S AUREUS IN AD

It is known that more than 90% of AD patients are colonized with S aureus, as compared with only 10% in healthy individuals.[38] The severity of dermatitis correlates with the density of S aureus colonization on AD skin lesions.[39] Anti–S aureus antibiotics have been shown to improve the severity of AD.[40] These observations have provided support for the role of S aureus in the pathogenesis of AD. Deficiency in AMP expression suggests an intrinsic defect in the innate immunity of AD.[41] S aureus is detected by pattern-recognition receptors in the innate immune system. Among the best-studied pattern-recognition receptors are the Toll-like receptors (TLRs). TLR2 has been associated with the recognition of the cell wall components (lipoteichoic acid and possibly peptidoglycan) of gram-positive bacteria including S aureus.[42] Ahmad-Nejad and colleagues[43] showed that TLR2 polymorphism R735Q is associated with a subgroup of patients with severe AD. Using human embryonic kidney 293 transfection system, they showed that this TLR2 polymorphism is associated with a significantly decreased expression of nuclear factor (NF)-κB, interferon-inducible protein 10, and IL-8.[44] TLR2-mediated production of IL-8 was shown to be significantly decreased in the monocytes of AD patients with TLR2 R735Q polymorphism.[44] On the other hand, the monocytes of these patients express significantly higher levels of IL-6 and IL-12 when compared with AD patients with wild-type TLR2.[45] Hasannejad and colleagues[46] showed that TLR2-mediated production of IL-1β and tumor necrosis factor-α by monocytes was significantly diminished in AD patients. Dysregulation of cytokine production as a result of TLR defects may lead to inflammation in AD.[45] More recently, another TLR2 polymorphism, A-16934 T, has also been associated with severe AD.[47]

In addition to the cell wall components of S aureus, alpha toxin from this bacterium is also capable of inducing immune dysregulation in AD. The prevalence of alpha toxin–producing S aureus strains isolated from AD patients ranges from 30% to 60%,[48,49] and the presence of alpha toxin–producing S aureus is significantly associated with extrinsic AD.[48] Alpha toxin was found to induce profound keratinocyte cytotoxicity and lymphocyte apoptosis.[49,50] It also activates T cells to produce interferon (IFN)-γ, leading to the development of chronic AD.[49] Other staphylococcal products that are frequently implicated in the pathogenesis of AD are their enterotoxins (superantigens).

THE ROLE OF STAPHYLOCOCCAL SUPERANTIGENS IN AD

Superantigens are presented on the MHC II molecules of antigen-presenting cells to activate T cells. These antigens bind directly to the common variable β (vβ) chains of T-cell receptors, resulting in a polyclonal activation of T cells. Classical staphylococcal enterotoxins include staphylococcal enterotoxin (SE) A, SEB, SEC, SED, and toxic shock syndrome toxin-1 (TSST-1). About 50% of S aureus isolated from AD patients secrete superantigens.[51–53] Direct application of superantigen on normal skin and unaffected AD skin induces erythema and causes flaring of skin disease in AD patients.[54] Increased AD severity correlates with the presence of superantigen-producing S aureus.[53,55] Skin biopsy studies have shown the presence of vβ T-cell clones corresponding to the specific superantigens in the AD lesions.[52] SEB has also been shown to induce lymphocyte expression of IL-31,[56] and this correlates with increased severity of AD.[57] A recent study that included classical and nonclassical staphylococcal superantigens (SEE and SEG-SEQ) showed that at least 80% of S aureus isolated from AD patients are superantigen-producing.[58] Of these patients, a median number of 8 different superantigens were found per S aureus isolate.[58,59] Patients with severe, corticosteroid-insensitive AD have been reported to harbor S aureus strains that produce significantly higher number of superantigens per organism, as compared with that in a general population of AD patients.[59] These S aureus strains that produce multiple superantigens, including SEB, SEC, TSST-1, and SEI-Q, are also associated with methicillin-resistant S aureus (MRSA),[5] which may be a complicating factor in moderate to severe AD.[60]

In addition to their ability to directly activate T cells, staphylococcal superantigens also induce the production of superantigen-specific IgE in AD patients.[61] Sensitization to superantigen-specific IgE has been correlated with the severity of AD.[62] The prevalence of superantigen-specific IgE in varying AD severity is as follows: 50% to 80% in severe AD,[51,61] 60% in moderate AD, and 40% in mild AD patients,[63] as compared with none in healthy individuals.[61] Binding of superantigen-specific IgE with respective superantigen leads to the activation of basophils,[61] which may play a crucial role in the initiation of IgE-mediated inflammation.[64]

THE ROLE OF VIRAL SKIN INFECTIONS IN AD

AD patients are also susceptible to viral skin infection.[22] EH, which is caused by HSV, can present as a life-threatening infection. AD patients with disseminated EH present with fever, malaise, and generalized vesicles.[3] EH patients may develop complications including keratoconjunctivitis, viremia, meningitis, encephalitis, or secondary bacterial sepsis. Another life-threatening viral infection that may occur in AD is eczema vaccinatum (EV), which is caused by vaccinia virus in smallpox vaccine. Since the eradication of smallpox virus in the early seventies, routine vaccination with vaccinia viruses (VV) had been discontinued in the general population in 1972 and in military personnel in 1990. However, because of bioterrorism threats in recent years, a government program to vaccinate select military personnel and public health workers with smallpox vaccine has been reinstituted. Since then, one case of EV has been reported in the United States. An infant with AD contracted EV through his father, who was in the military and had received smallpox vaccine 21 days before the onset of the infant's symptoms.[65] The infant needed life-saving measures including the use of investigational drugs via Emergency Investigational New Drug Application. The case illustrates the importance of understanding the mechanisms of VV infection in AD to identify AD patients at high risk for EV and to devise new treatments in AD patients with EV. Because of the rarity of EV and its clinical resemblance to EH,[65,66] understanding the mechanism of disease in EH has proven to be fruitful.

Beck and colleagues,[67] in the National Institute of Allergy and Infectious Diseases-funded multicenter Atopic Dermatitis and Vaccinia Network (ADVN) study, have recently shown that a subgroup of AD patients is particularly susceptible to EH. This subgroup has more severe disease, a higher number of circulating eosinophils, higher levels of serum CCL17, more asthma, and specific IgE sensitization to inhaled and food allergens as compared with AD patients with no history of EH. Patients with history of EH are also more likely to have secondary skin infections with S aureus. The clinical observation that patients with extrinsic AD are more susceptible to viral infection is consistent with laboratory findings that IL-4 and IL-13 suppress keratinocyte expression of the cathelicidin AMP, LL-37, which has potent antiviral activity against HSV or VV.[68,69] Viral infections in AD further trigger the production of TSLP via TLR3, which increases the Th2 cytokine milieu in AD lesions, thereby leading to further susceptibility to disseminated viral infections.[70] IL-4 and IL-13 have also been found to suppress the expression of S100 calcium-binding protein A11 (S100A11) in keratinocytes.[71] Suppression of S100A11 expression leads to the down-regulation of IL-10R2, which is a receptor for IFN-λ, a cytokine with activity against VV.[72]

Gao and colleagues[73] showed that a history of EH in AD patients was significantly associated with FLG mutations. The frequency of R501X FLG was 3 times higher in AD patients with EH as compared with those without EH. These findings were seen in European and African Americans.[73] More recently, microarray analyses were applied to study VV-induced transcriptional changes in unaffected skin explants obtained from AD, psoriatic, and healthy individuals.[74] The skin samples were treated in vitro with vehicle or VV and subjected to gene ontology analysis. Wound healing and defense response genes were found to be among the most affected genes in AD-specific responses to VV. Innate immunity genes, including leukotriene B4 receptor (LTB4R), orosomucoid 1 (ORM1), coagulation factor II (thrombin) receptor (F2R), complement component 9 (C9), and lipopolysaccharide binding protein (LBP), were found to be significantly down-regulated in VV-treated AD explants, as compared with healthy individuals or psoriasis patients. These observations were confirmed with real-time polymerase chain reaction (PCR). In addition, the down-regulation of innate immune response gene ORM1, TLR4, and NACHT leucine-rich repeat protein 1 (NLRP1) were found to be associated with AD severity. The last 2 genes, TLR4 and NLRP1, are cell surface and intracellular pattern-recognition receptors, respectively, for microbial pathogens.

Compared with chronic AD lesions, acute AD lesions have been shown to have increased expression of IL-17.[75,76] Patera and colleagues[77] first noted that IL-17 increased the virulence of VV. In an AD mouse model, increased IL-17 expression was found to be associated with filaggrin-deficient mice[78] and was responsible for the dissemination of VV in AD lesions.[79] This effect of IL-17 may be caused by its suppression of NK activity against VV.[80]

THE ROLE OF FUNGI IN AD

The role of fungi in AD has been based primarily on observations of colonization by *Malassezia* species in AD patients. There has been controversy whether AD patients have increased colonization with *Malassezia* species as compared with healthy controls. The controversy stems from differences in sampling methods, culture techniques, and identification of different species. Using molecular techniques (nested and real-time PCR), Sugita and colleagues[81] found that *Malassezia* colonization is common in AD patients and healthy subjects, with detection rates of 100% and 78%, respectively. Among the AD patients, these investigators found that the head and neck areas are 7 and 10 times more likely to be colonized with *Malassezia* than the limb and trunk areas, respectively.[82]

Baroni and colleagues[83] found that *Malassezia furfur* may induce AMP and IL-8 expression in keratinocytes via TLR2. Selander and colleagues[84] found both TLR2-independent and -dependent pathways in the activation of mast cells by *Malassezia sympodialis*. These investigators showed that *M sympodialis* induced the release of cysteinyl leukotrienes from non-IgE–sensitized mast cells. Using knockout mice for TLR2 and MyD88, an adaptor molecule in most TLR pathways, they showed that IgE-sensitized mast cell degranulation and release of the chemokine MCP-1 was independent of TLR2 and MyD88, whereas IL-6 production was dependent on the TLR2/MyD88 pathway.[84] These findings are consistent with a recent study that showed the importance of a non-TLR pattern-recognition receptor, Mincle, in the recognition of *Malassezia* by the host immune system.[85] In that study, *Malassezia* was shown to activate inflammatory responses in macrophages via Mincle.[85]

Malassezia species also induce the production of *Malassezia*-specific IgE in AD patients. These specific IgE sensitizations were found exclusively in AD patients, but not in patients with allergic rhinitis, urticaria, or allergic contact dermatitis.[86] *Malassezia*-specific IgE molecules are significantly more prevalent in AD patients with head and neck dermatitis, as compared with AD patients with lesions in other locations (100% vs 14%).[87] The prevalence and degree of IgE sensitization to *Malassezia* in AD patients are also age- and severity-dependent. Adult AD patients were found to have higher specific IgE levels of *Malassezia* than children with AD.[88] Among young children with AD, the prevalence of IgE sensitization to *Malassezia* were also significantly higher in the older age group than in infants.[89] However, infants with severe AD and repeated oozing lesions are particularly at risk for developing specific IgE against *Malassezia*.[90]

Malassezia may also contribute to AD inflammation via cell-mediated immunity and IgE-mediated autoimmunity. Patients with intrinsic AD were also found to have a significantly higher prevalence of positive atopy patch tests to *M sympodialis* as compared with healthy controls (38% vs 0%).[86,91] IgE-binding epitopes from *M sympodialis* may cross-react with the human IgE autoantigen, manganese superoxide dismutase.[92] This may explain the ability of human manganese superoxide dismutase in inducing eczematous reactions in *M sympodialis*–sensitized patients.[93]

THE ROLE OF OTHER MICROBIAL PATHOGENS IN AD

Group A beta hemolytic *Streptococcus* also causes skin infections in AD.[94] Streptococcal infection is associated with severe AD[95] and may result in complications including acute poststreptococcal glomerulonephritis, hypertension, and posterior reversible encephalopathy syndrome.[96] Molluscum contagiosum (MC) virus belongs to the family of poxviruses. MC causes skin lesions characterized by flesh-colored papules. AD patients are at increased risk for having a higher number of MC lesions.[97] In addition, these lesions may lead to disfiguring scars in AD patients.[98] Patients with EH are also at increased risk for MC.[67]

CLINICAL IMPLICATIONS

The discovery of FLG mutations as a predisposing factor for AD may lead to a new molecular classification of eczema. Although it has been shown that FLG facilitates the production of IgE in a mouse model of FLG mutation, whether FLG plays a role in modifying the immune response of AD in humans remains to be proven. Further understanding of FLG function may result in the development of targeted therapy in AD, for example by increasing the expression of filaggrin.[99] Not only will this approach help AD patients with their skin disease, it may prevent the development of asthma in these patients because multiple studies have now confirmed the association of asthma with FLG mutations in such patients. Genetic polymorphisms in the immune system remain an important area of research in the pathogenesis of AD. Increasing evidence suggests that innate immunity is the primary driver of adaptive immunity. Genetic polymorphisms in TLR2, which is the chief extracellular pattern-recognition receptor for *S aureus*, illustrates the potential role of innate immunity in defining the phenotypes of AD. These findings are crucial because *S aureus* cell wall products have now been shown to be capable of enhancing the production of TSLP, a key molecule in subsequent Th2 immune responses, which include the production of IL-4 and IL-13. The roles of these 2 cytokines in AD have been well characterized; they have been shown to suppress the expression of AMPs, filaggrin, and S100A11, all of which contribute to the pathogenesis of AD. Therefore, IL-4 and IL-13 remain important targets in therapy for AD. The pathogenic roles of *S aureus* in AD are numerous, including the production of superantigens, alpha toxin, stimulation of host TLR, and superantigen-specific IgE. Because chronic use of antibiotics leads to the development of resistant bacteria such as MRSA, which has an emerging role in AD, new therapeutic approaches against *S aureus* in AD are needed.[1] A recent study showed that bleach baths lead to significant improvement of AD in children, although patients remain colonized by *S aureus*.[100] Useful information on the role of viral infections in AD has been generated by ADVN studies. The identification of the subgroup of AD patients with increased susceptibility to EH, that is, those with more severe disease, early age of onset, increased Th2 response, and allergic sensitization to common allergens, may help identify those AD patients who are at highest risk for EV. These observations may help clinicians in weighing the risks and benefits of smallpox vaccine in AD patients, if the threat of bioterrorism with smallpox becomes imminent. Direct studies of VV infection in in vitro or mouse models have also helped to elucidate the mechanisms of VV infection in AD. The studies by Bin and colleagues[72] and Grigoryev and colleagues[74] provide further insight into the genes that are critical for the innate immune responses against VV. These insights in turn may lead to novel approaches in treating or preventing VV infection in AD, for example, up-regulation of S100A11, IL-10R2, ORM1, TLR4, or NLRP1 to increase innate immune response against VV. Increased expression of IL-17 in acute AD lesions may be an important predisposing factor in AD patients' susceptibility to VV. Thus, IL-17 may be a therapeutic target in limiting VV dissemination in AD patients. Because *Malassezia* species play an important pathogenic role in a subgroup of AD patients, the identification of Mincle as the host pattern-recognition receptor for *Malassezia* may lead to novel therapies against this pathogen in AD.

REFERENCES

1. Boguniewicz M, Leung DY. Recent insights into atopic dermatitis and implications for management of infectious complications. J Allergy Clin Immunol 2010;125:4–13.
2. Benenson S, Zimhony O, Dahan D, et al. Atopic dermatitis—a risk factor for invasive *Staphylococcus aureus* infections: two cases and review. Am J Med 2005;118:1048–51.
3. Wollenberg A, Wetzel S, Burgdorf WH, et al. Viral infections in atopic dermatitis: pathogenic aspects and clinical management. J Allergy Clin Immunol 2003; 112(4):667–74.
4. O'Regan GM, Sandilands A, McLean WH, et al. Filaggrin in atopic dermatitis. J Allergy Clin Immunol 2009;124(3 Suppl 2):R2–6.
5. Schlievert PM, Strandberg KL, Lin YC, et al. Secreted virulence factor comparison between methicillin-resistant and methicillin-sensitive *Staphylococcus aureus*, and its relevance to atopic dermatitis. J Allergy Clin Immunol 2010; 125:39–49.
6. Grice K, Sattar H, Baker H, et al. The relationship of transepidermal water loss to skin temperature in psoriasis and eczema. J Invest Dermatol 1975;64(5):313–5.
7. Seidenari S, Giusti G. Objective assessment of the skin of children affected by atopic dermatitis: a study of pH, capacitance and TEWL in eczematous and clinically uninvolved skin. Acta Derm Venereol 1995;75(6):429–33.
8. Cork MJ, Robinson DA, Vasilopoulos Y, et al. New perspectives on epidermal barrier dysfunction in atopic dermatitis: gene-environment interactions. J Allergy Clin Immunol 2006;118(1):3–21.
9. Gupta J, Grube E, Ericksen MB, et al. Intrinsically defective skin barrier function in children with atopic dermatitis correlates with disease severity. J Allergy Clin Immunol 2008;121(3):725–30.
10. Jensen JM, Fölster-Holst R, Baranowsky A, et al. Impaired sphingomyelinase activity and epidermal differentiation in atopic dermatitis. J Invest Dermatol 2004;122(6):1423–31.
11. Elias PM, Hatano Y, Williams ML. Basis for the barrier abnormality in atopic dermatitis: outside-inside-outside pathogenic mechanisms. J Allergy Clin Immunol 2008;121(6):1337–43.
12. Stemmler S, Parwez Q, Petrasch-Parwez E, et al. Two common loss-of-function mutations within the filaggrin gene predispose for early onset of atopic dermatitis. J Invest Dermatol 2007;127(3):722–4.
13. Brown SJ, Sandilands A, Zhao Y, et al. Prevalent and low-frequency null mutations in the filaggrin gene are associated with early-onset and persistent atopic eczema. J Invest Dermatol 2008;128(6):1591–4.

14. Barker JN, Palmer CN, Zhao Y, et al. Null mutations in the filaggrin gene (FLG) determine major susceptibility to early-onset atopic dermatitis that persists into adulthood. J Invest Dermatol 2007;127(3):564–7.
15. Weidinger S, Rodriguez E, Stahl C, et al. Filaggrin mutations strongly predispose to early-onset and extrinsic atopic dermatitis. J Invest Dermatol 2007; 127(3):724–6.
16. Weidinger S, Illig T, Baurecht H, et al. Loss-of-function variations within the filaggrin gene predispose for atopic dermatitis with allergic sensitizations. J Allergy Clin Immunol 2006;118(1):214–9.
17. Marenholz I, Nickel R, Ruschendorf F, et al. Filaggrin loss-of-function mutations predispose to phenotypes involved in the atopic march. J Allergy Clin Immunol 2006;118(4):866–71.
18. Henderson J, Northstone K, Lee SP, et al. The burden of disease associated with filaggrin mutations: a population-based, longitudinal birth cohort study. J Allergy Clin Immunol 2008;121(4):872–7.
19. Rogers AJ, Celedon JC, Lasky-Su JA, et al. Filaggrin mutations confer susceptibility to atopic dermatitis but not to asthma. J Allergy Clin Immunol 2007; 120(6):1332–7.
20. Fallon PG, Sasaki T, Sandilands A, et al. A homozygous frameshift mutation in the mouse Flg gene facilitates enhanced percutaneous allergen priming. Nat Genet 2009;41:602–8.
21. Smith FJ, Irvine AD, Terron-Kwiatkowski A, et al. Loss-of-function mutations in the gene encoding filaggrin cause ichthyosis vulgaris. Nat Genet 2006;38(3):337–42.
22. Christophers E, Henseler T. Contrasting disease patterns in psoriasis and atopic dermatitis. Arch Dermatol Res 1987;279(Suppl):S48–51.
23. Arikawa J, Ishibashi M, Kawashima M, et al. Decreased levels of sphingosine, a natural antimicrobial agent, may be associated with vulnerability of the stratum corneum from patients with atopic dermatitis to colonization by Staphylococcus aureus. J Invest Dermatol 2002;119(2):433–9.
24. Rieg S, Steffen H, Seeber S, et al. Deficiency of dermcidin-derived antimicrobial peptides in sweat of patients with atopic dermatitis correlates with an impaired innate defense of human skin in vivo. J Immunol 2005;174(12):8003–10.
25. Ong PY, Ohtake T, Brandt C, et al. Endogenous antimicrobial peptides and skin infections in atopic dermatitis. N Engl J Med 2002;347:1151–60.
26. Nomura I, Goleva E, Howell MD, et al. Cytokine milieu of atopic dermatitis, as compared to psoriasis, skin prevents induction of innate immune response genes. J Immunol 2003;171:3262–9.
27. Allakhverdi Z, Comeau MR, Jessup HK, et al. Thymic stromal lymphopoietin is released by human epithelial cells in response to microbes, trauma, or inflammation and potently activates mast cells. J Exp Med 2007;204:253–8.
28. Cho SH, Strickland I, Tomkinson A, et al. Preferential binding of Staphylococcus aureus to skin sites of Th2-mediated inflammation in a murine model. J Invest Dermatol 2001;116:658–63.
29. Howell MD, Kim BE, Gao P, et al. Cytokine modulation of atopic dermatitis filaggrin skin expression. J Allergy Clin Immunol 2009;124(3 Suppl 2):R7–12.
30. Kisich KO, Carspecken CW, Fiéve S, et al. Defective killing of Staphylococcus aureus in atopic dermatitis is associated with reduced mobilization of human beta-defensin-3. J Allergy Clin Immunol 2008;122(1):62–8.
31. Liang SC, Tan XY, Luxenberg DP, et al. Interleukin (IL)-22 and IL-17 are coexpressed by Th17 cells and cooperatively enhance expression of antimicrobial peptides. J Exp Med 2006;203(10):2271–9.

32. Guttman-Yassky E, Lowes MA, Fuentes-Duculan J, et al. Low expression of the IL-23/Th17 pathway in atopic dermatitis compared to psoriasis. J Immunol 2008; 181(10):7420–7.

33. Eyerich K, Pennino D, Scarponi C, et al. IL-17 in atopic eczema: linking allergen-specific adaptive and microbial-triggered innate immune response. J Allergy Clin Immunol 2009;123(1):59–66, e4.

34. Leung AD, Schiltz AM, Hall CF, et al. Severe atopic dermatitis is associated with a high burden of environmental *Staphylococcus aureus*. Clin Exp Allergy 2008; 38(5):789–93.

35. Bonness S, Szekat C, Novak N, et al. Pulsed-field gel electrophoresis of *Staphylococcus aureus* isolates from atopic patients revealing presence of similar strains in isolates from children and their parents. J Clin Microbiol 2008;46: 456–61.

36. Chiu LS, Ho MS, Hsu LY, et al. Prevalence and molecular characteristics of *Staphylococcus aureus* isolates colonizing patients with atopic dermatitis and their close contacts in Singapore. Br J Dermatol 2009;160(5):965–71.

37. Gilani SJ, Gonzalez M, Hussain I, et al. *Staphylococcus aureus* re-colonization in atopic dermatitis: beyond the skin. Clin Exp Dermatol 2005;30:10–3.

38. Leyden JJ, Marples RR, Kligman AM. *Staphylococcus aureus* in the lesions of atopic dermatitis. Br J Dermatol 1974;90:525–30.

39. Williams RE, Gibson AG, Aitchison TC, et al. Assessment of a contact-plate sampling technique and subsequent quantitative bacterial studies in atopic dermatitis. Br J Dermatol 1990;123(4):493–501.

40. Breuer K, HAussler S, Kapp A, et al. *Staphylococcus aureus*: colonizing features and influence of an antibacterial treatment in adults with atopic dermatitis. Br J Dermatol 2002;147(1):55–61.

41. Ong PY. Is/are pattern recognition receptor(s) for *Staphylococcus aureus* defective in atopic dermatitis? Dermatology 2006;212(1):19–22.

42. Fournier B, Philpott DJ. Recognition of *Staphylococcus aureus* by the innate immune system. Clin Microbiol Rev 2005;18(3):521–40.

43. Ahmad-Nejad P, Mrabet-Dahbi S, Breuer K, et al. The toll-like receptor 2 R753Q polymorphism defines a subgroup of patients with atopic dermatitis having severe phenotype. J Allergy Clin Immunol 2004;113:565–7.

44. Mrabet-Dahbi S, Dalpke AH, Niebuhr M, et al. The Toll-like receptor 2 R753Q mutation modifies cytokine production and Toll-like receptor expression in atopic dermatitis. J Allergy Clin Immunol 2008;121(4):1013–9.

45. Niebuhr M, Langnickel J, Draing C, et al. Dysregulation of toll-like receptor-2 (TLR-2)-induced effects in monocytes from patients with atopic dermatitis: impact of the TLR-2 R753Q polymorphism. Allergy 2008;63(6):728–34.

46. Hasannejad H, Takahashi R, Kimishima M, et al. Selective impairment of Toll-like receptor 2-mediated proinflammatory cytokine production by monocytes from patients with atopic dermatitis. J Allergy Clin Immunol 2007;120(1):69–75.

47. Oh DY, Schumann RR, Hamann L, et al. Association of the toll-like receptor 2 A-16934T promoter polymorphism with severe atopic dermatitis. Allergy 2009; 64(11):1608–15.

48. Wichmann K, Uter W, Weiss J, et al. Isolation of alpha-toxin-producing *Staphylococcus aureus* from the skin of highly sensitized adult patients with severe atopic dermatitis. Br J Dermatol 2009;161(2):300–5.

49. Breuer K, Wittmann M, Kempe K, et al. Alpha-toxin is produced by skin colonizing *Staphylococcus aureus* and induces a T helper type 1 response in atopic dermatitis. Clin Exp Allergy 2005;35:1088–95.

50. Ezepchuk YV, Leung DY, Middleton MH, et al. Staphylococcal toxins and protein A differentially induce cytotoxicity and release of tumor necrosis factor-alpha from human keratinocytes. J Invest Dermatol 1996;107:603–9.
51. Nomura I, Tanaka K, Tomita H, et al. Evaluation of the staphylococcal exotoxins and their specific IgE in childhood atopic dermatitis. J Allergy Clin Immunol 1999;104:441–6.
52. Bunikowski R, Mielke ME, Skarabis H, et al. Evidence for a disease-promoting effect of *Staphylococcus aureus*-derived exotoxins in atopic dermatitis. J Allergy Clin Immunol 2000;105:814–9.
53. Tomi NS, Kranke B, Aberer E. Staphylococcal toxins in patients with psoriasis, atopic dermatitis, and erythroderma, and in healthy control subjects. J Am Acad Dermatol 2005;53:67–72.
54. Strange P, Skov L, Lisby S, et al. Staphylococcal enterotoxin B applied on intact normal and intact atopic skin induces dermatitis. Arch Dermatol 1996;132(1): 27–33.
55. Zollner TM, Wichelhaus TA, Hartung A, et al. Colonization with superantigen-producing *Staphylococcus aureus* is associated with increased severity of atopic dermatitis. Clin Exp Allergy 2000;30:994–1000.
56. Sonkoly E, Muller A, Lauerma AI, et al. IL-31: a new link between T cells and pruritus in atopic skin inflammation. J Allergy Clin Immunol 2006;117(2):411–7.
57. Raap U, Wichmann K, Bruder M, et al. Correlation of IL-31 serum levels with severity of atopic dermatitis. J Allergy Clin Immunol 2008;122(2):421–3.
58. Leung DY, Hanifin JM, Pariser DM, et al. Effects of pimecrolimus cream 1% in the treatment of patients with atopic dermatitis who demonstrate a clinical insensitivity to topical corticosteroids: a randomized, multicentre vehicle-controlled trial. Br J Dermatol 2009;161(2):435–43.
59. Schlievert PM, Case LC, Strandberg KL, et al. Superantigen profile of *Staphylococcus aureus* isolates from patients with steroid-resistant atopic dermatitis. Clin Infect Dis 2008;46:1562–7.
60. Hon KL, Leung AK, Kong AY, et al. Atopic dermatitis complicated by methicillin-resistant *Staphylococcus aureus* infection. J Natl Med Assoc 2008;100(7): 797–800.
61. Leung DYM, Harbeck R, Bina P, et al. Presence of IgE antibodies to staphylococcal exotoxins on the skin of patients with atopic dermatitis. Evidence for a new group of allergens. J Clin Invest 1993;92:1374–80.
62. Bunikowski R, Mielke M, Skarabis H, et al. Prevalence and role of serum IgE antibodies to the *Staphylococcus aureus*-derived superantigens SEA and SEB in children with atopic dermatitis. J Allergy Clin Immunol 1999;103(1 Pt 1):119–24.
63. Ong PY, Patel M, Ferdman RM, et al. Association of staphylococcal superantigen-specific immunoglobulin e with mild and moderate atopic dermatitis. J Pediatr 2008;153(6):803–6.
64. Karasuyama H, Mukai K, Tsujimura Y, et al. Newly discovered roles for basophils: a neglected minority gains new respect. Nat Rev Immunol 2009;9(1):9–13.
65. Vora S, Damon I, Fulginiti V, et al. Severe eczema vaccinatum in a household contact of a smallpox vaccinee. Clin Infect Dis 2008;46(10):1555–61.
66. Boyd DA, Sperling LC, Norton SA. Eczema herpeticum and clinical criteria for investigating smallpox. Emerg Infect Dis 2009;15(7):1102–4.
67. Beck LA, Boguniewicz M, Hata T, et al. Phenotype of atopic dermatitis subjects with a history of eczema herpeticum. J Allergy Clin Immunol 2009;124(2):260–9.
68. Howell MD, Wollenberg A, Gallo RL, et al. Cathelicidin deficiency predisposes to eczema herpeticum. J Allergy Clin Immunol 2006;117(4):836–41.

69. Howell MD, Gallo RL, Boguniewicz M, et al. Cytokine milieu of atopic dermatitis skin subverts the innate immune response to vaccinia virus. Immunity 2006; 24(3):341–8.

70. Kinoshita H, Takai T, Le TA, et al. Cytokine milieu modulates release of thymic stromal lymphopoietin from human keratinocytes stimulated with double-stranded RNA. J Allergy Clin Immunol 2009;123(1):179–86.

71. Howell MD, Fairchild HR, Kim BE, et al. Th2 cytokines act on S100/A11 to down-regulate keratinocyte differentiation. J Invest Dermatol 2008;128(9):2248–58.

72. Bin L, Howell MD, Kim BE, et al. Inhibition of S100A11 gene expression impairs keratinocyte response against vaccinia virus through downregulation of the IL-10 receptor 2 chain. J Allergy Clin Immunol 2009;124(2):270–7.

73. Gao PS, Rafaels NM, Hand T, et al. Filaggrin mutations that confer risk of atopic dermatitis confer greater risk for eczema herpeticum. J Allergy Clin Immunol 2009;124(3):507–13.

74. Grigoryev DN, Howell MD, Watkins TN, et al. Vaccinia virus-specific molecular signature in atopic dermatitis skin. J Allergy Clin Immunol 2010;125: 153–9, e28.

75. Toda M, Leung DY, Molet S, et al. Polarized in vivo expression of IL-11 and IL-17 between acute and chronic skin lesions. J Allergy Clin Immunol 2003;111(4): 875–81.

76. Koga C, Kabashima K, Shiraishi N, et al. Possible pathogenic role of Th17 cells for atopic dermatitis. J Invest Dermatol 2008;128(11):2625–30.

77. Patera AC, Pesnicak L, Bertin J, et al. Interleukin 17 modulates the immune response to vaccinia virus infection. Virology 2002;299(1):56–63.

78. Oyoshi MK, Murphy GF, Geha RS. Filaggrin-deficient mice exhibit TH17-dominated skin inflammation and permissiveness to epicutaneous sensitization with protein antigen. J Allergy Clin Immunol 2009;124(3):485–93.

79. Oyoshi MK, Elkhal A, Kumar L, et al. Vaccinia virus inoculation in sites of allergic skin inflammation elicits a vigorous cutaneous IL-17 response. Proc Natl Acad Sci U S A 2009;106(35):14954–9.

80. Kawakami Y, Tomimori Y, Yumoto K, et al. Inhibition of NK cell activity by IL-17 allows vaccinia virus to induce severe skin lesions in a mouse model of eczema vaccinatum. J Exp Med 2009;206(6):1219–25.

81. Sugita T, Suto H, Unno T, et al. Molecular analysis of Malassezia microflora on the skin of atopic dermatitis patients and healthy subjects. J Clin Microbiol 2001;39(10):3486–90.

82. Sugita T, Tajima M, Tsubuku H, et al. Quantitative analysis of cutaneous Malassezia in atopic dermatitis patients using real-time PCR. Microbiol Immunol 2006; 50(7):549–52.

83. Baroni A, Orlando M, Donnarumma G, et al. Toll-like receptor 2 (TLR2) mediates intracellular signalling in human keratinocytes in response to Malassezia furfur. Arch Dermatol Res 2006;297(7):280–8.

84. Selander C, Engblom C, Nilsson G, et al. TLR2/MyD88-dependent and -independent activation of mast cell IgE responses by the skin commensal yeast Malassezia sympodialis. J Immunol 2009;182(7):4208–16.

85. Yamasaki S, Matsumoto M, Takeuchi O, et al. C-type lectin Mincle is an activating receptor for pathogenic fungus, Malassezia. Proc Natl Acad Sci U S A 2009;106(6):1897–902.

86. Casagrande BF, Flückiger S, Linder MT, et al. Sensitization to the yeast Malassezia sympodialis is specific for extrinsic and intrinsic atopic eczema. J Invest Dermatol 2006;126(11):2414–21.

87. Devos SA, van der Valk PG. The relevance of skin prick tests for *Pityrosporum ovale* in patients with head and neck dermatitis. Allergy 2000;55(11):1056–8.
88. Takahata Y, Sugita T, Kato H, et al. Cutaneous Malassezia flora in atopic dermatitis differs between adults and children. Br J Dermatol 2007;157(6):1178–82.
89. Ong PY, Ferdman RM, Church JA. Late-onset of IgE sensitization to microbial allergens in young children with atopic dermatitis. Br J Dermatol 2010;162(1): 159–61.
90. Lange L, Alter N, Keller T, et al. Sensitization to Malassezia in infants and children with atopic dermatitis: prevalence and clinical characteristics. Allergy 2008;63(4):486–7.
91. Johansson C, Sandström MH, Bartosik J, et al. Atopy patch test reactions to Malassezia allergens differentiate subgroups of atopic dermatitis patients. Br J Dermatol 2003;148(3):479–88.
92. Vilhelmsson M, Glaser AG, Martinez DB, et al. Mutational analysis of amino acid residues involved in IgE-binding to the *Malassezia sympodialis* allergen Mala s 11. Mol Immunol 2008;46(2):294–303.
93. Schmid-Grendelmeier P, Flückiger S, Disch R, et al. IgE-mediated and T cell-mediated autoimmunity against manganese superoxide dismutase in atopic dermatitis. J Allergy Clin Immunol 2005;115(5):1068–75.
94. Brook I, Frazier EH, Yeager JK. Microbiology of infected atopic dermatitis. Int J Dermatol 1996;35(11):791–3.
95. Hayakawa K, Hirahara K, Fukuda T, et al. Risk factors for severe impetiginized atopic dermatitis in Japan and assessment of its microbiological features. Clin Exp Dermatol 2009;34(5):e63–5.
96. Park JM, Oh SH, Kim J, et al. Atopic dermatitis with group A beta-hemolytic Streptococcus skin infection complicated by posterior reversible encephalopathy syndrome. Arch Dermatol 2009;145(7):846–7.
97. Dohil MA, Lin P, Lee J, et al. The epidemiology of molluscum contagiosum in children. J Am Acad Dermatol 2006;54(1):47–54.
98. Ghura HS, Camp RD. Scarring molluscum contagiosum in patients with severe atopic dermatitis: report of two cases. Br J Dermatol 2001;144(5):1094–5.
99. Sandilands A, Sutherland C, Irvine AD, et al. Filaggrin in the frontline: role in skin barrier function and disease. J Cell Sci 2009;122(Pt 9):1285–94.
100. Huang JT, Abrams M, Tlougan B, et al. Treatment of *Staphylococcus aureus* colonization in atopic dermatitis decreases disease severity. Pediatrics 2009; 123(5):e808–14.

Atopic Dermatitis and Keratoconjunctivitis

Brett Bielory, MD[a], Leonard Bielory, MD[b,c],*

KEYWORDS

- Atopic dermatitis • Atopic keratoconjunctivitis • Ocular allergy
- Blepharoconjunctivitis • Keratoconus

Atopic keratoconjunctivitis (AKC) is a more common chronic inflammatory disorder of the eye than previously appreciated. It is a potentially blinding ocular condition with disabling symptomatology because it involves inflammation of the cornea ("kerato") and the conjunctiva. In 1952, Hogan[1,2] first described AKC as a bilateral conjunctivitis occurring in five male patients with atopic dermatitis (AD). Other atopic ocular disorders include seasonal and perennial allergic conjunctivitis, giant papillary conjunctivitis, and vernal conjunctivitis (**Box 1**).[3,4]

IMMUNOPATHOPHYSIOLOGY

The histopathologic findings of AKC are diagnostically specific and include a mixture of mast cell, eosinophil, and lymphocyte infiltration into the conjunctival epithelium that seems to be a hybrid of Th1 and Th2 interactions.[5] This is further supported by in situ hybridization studies of ocular tissue showing increased levels of mRNA for interleukin (IL)-3, -4, and -5 compared with normal tissue. IL-2 and -5 mRNA expression have been found to be significantly higher in subjects with AKC, as have IL-4 tear levels.[6] In addition, interferon (IFN)-γ mRNA expression was greater in patients with AKC than in control subjects ($P = .005$).[7] The increased IFN-γ significantly correlated with corneal involvement, a sign of disease severity, and upregulated intercellular adhesion molecule-1 on conjunctival fibroblasts.[6] Overall, AKC seems to have a slight

Financial disclosures: B. Bielory has nothing to disclose. L. Bielory has received financial support from Schering-Plough, Glaxo-Smith-Kline, Merck, Otsuka, Novartis, Sanofi-Aventis, Genentech, Astellas, UCB-Pharma, Alcon, Meda, Inspire, Santen, Allergan, ISTA, SARCode, Bausch and Lomb, Vistakon, ViroPharm, Dyax, Jerini, Ocusense (Tear Lab), and Rutgers University Press. No funding support was provided for the development of this article.

[a] Department of Ophthalmology, Bascom Palmer Eye Institute, University of Miami Miller School of Medicine, 900 NW 17th Street, Miami, FL 33136, USA
[b] STARx Allergy and Asthma Center, 400 Mountain Avenue, Springfield, NJ 07081, USA
[c] Center for Environmental Prediction, Rutgers University, 14 College Farm Road, New Brunswick, NJ 08901–8551, USA
* Corresponding author. STARx Allergy and Asthma Center, 400 Mountain Avenue, Springfield, NJ 07081.
E-mail address: drlbielory@gmail.com

Box 1
History and physical components of AKC

History

Chronic or chronically relapsing atopic disease

- Dermatitis
- Asthma
- Rhinitis
- Conjunctivitis

Ocular symptoms with little or no seasonal variation (as opposed to vernal conjunctivitis, which is predominantly seen only in warm weather, especially along the Mediterranean Sea basin)

- Itching
- Tearing
- Ropy discharge
- Burning
- Photophobia
- Decreased vision

Physical

Periocular

- Dennie-Morgan folds (linear lid folds)
- Hertoghe sign (absence of lateral eyebrows)

Lids

- Thickening and tylosis, crusting, edema, fissures
- Ptosis
- Staphylococcal blepharitis

Conjunctiva

- Small- or medium-sized papillae
- Hyperemia, edema, excessive mucin
- Limbal Trantas dots (clusters of necrotic eosinophils, neutrophils, and epithelial cells)
- Formation of keratinization, cicatrization, and symblepharon in advanced disease

Cornea

- Punctate epitheliopathy and keratitis
- Persistent epithelial defects
- Shield-shaped ulcers
- Anterior stromal scarring
- Micropannus
- Extensive peripheral corneal vascularization in later stages
- Higher incidence of keratoconus (16%)
- Recurrent herpes simplex keratitis associated with AKC

Lens

- Anterior subcapsular shield-shaped cataracts
- Posterior cataracts (similar to steroid induced cataracts)

Fundus

- Degenerative vitreous changes
- Retinal detachment
- Uveitis (rare)

shift in mRNA expression to Th2-like T-cell cytokine profile.[7] In addition, tear fluid cytokines including IFN-γ, tumor necrosis factor-α, IL-2, IL-4, IL-5, and IL-10 levels seem to play an important pathophysiologic role in AKC.[8] IL-5 seems to correlate more closely with the proliferative forms of ocular allergy.[9]

CD4 lymphocytes are increased in various forms of chronic ocular allergy, such as AKC, and seem to require the P-selectin ligand for their direct infiltration into the conjunctiva.[10] Examining specific CD4 subsets, the percentages of naive Th (CD4/45RA+) and memory Th (CD4/29+) cells, and the Th/Ts and memory Th cells/naive Th cells ratios were measured in the blood and tear samples of patients with AKC, atopic patients without ocular involvement, and normal volunteers. The results showed that patients with AKC had significantly higher memory Th cell concentration especially in the tear samples, and Th/Ts and memory Th cells/naive Th cell ratios both in the tear and blood samples compared with normal subjects.[11] This further supports that the local ocular environment is important in the development of the more chronic forms of ocular disease, such as AKC. The complexities and the multicellular involvement continue to expand. Additional abnormalities, including conjunctival epithelium of patients with AD with Langerhans cells (CD1a+) bearing IgE on its surface, suggest that these cells may also be involved in eliciting the hypersensitivity reaction and may participate in ocular inflammation.[12–14]

A unique finding of the development of an AKC-like disease in four patients who had no history of atopic disorders and who received pluripotent hematopoietic stem cell replacement therapy has been reported, suggesting the potential of some form of adoptive transfer.[15]

The relationship of serum levels of IgE, LTB4, and food allergen sensitivity were significantly increased in AD patients with ocular complications compared with those without ocular complications.[16] In ocular-type AD, serum IgE was significantly increased in patients with cataracts compared with those without cataracts. In other studies, however, development of cataracts or retinal detachment had no relationship to serum IgE levels, personal history of respiratory atopy, the duration of topical corticosteroid use on the face, or treatment with systemic corticosteroids.[17] This suggests that patients who habitually rub their faces strongly tend to develop cataract or retinal detachment at a statistically significant higher frequency. Tear histamine and LTB4 levels in AD patients with ocular complications showed significant elevations compared with those in patients with pure AD and controls.[16]

Other mechanisms of corneal damage include eosinophilic activation and mediator release. There is evidence that sIgA secretion in the tears of patients with AD was significantly lower than that of normal subjects and a higher frequency of *Staphylococcus aureus* in the tears from patients with AD compared with normal subjects.[18] This suggests that the reduced sIgA secretion on the mucous membranes might play a crucial role in the pathogenesis of the ocular lesions. The common finding of *S aureus* colonization in AKC suggests a potential role for the activation of epithelial cells by Toll-like receptor 2 and the receptor for platelet-activating factor.[19] This is further supported in a mouse model of allergic conjunctivitis that demonstrated that inoculation of *S aureus* markedly accelerated the signs of allergic conjunctivitis and was associated with higher levels of IgE in serum. In addition, the mice inoculated with *S aureus* had more IL-4, IL-5, IL-13, and eotaxin secretion than the noninoculated group. In contrast, inoculation of Toll-like receptor 2 (−/−) mice with *S aureus* had no effect on severity of ocular symptoms. The findings further support that activation of Toll-like receptor 2 signaling by *S aureus* induces Th2-type immune responses and accelerates experimental allergic conjunctivitis.[20] Another issue is whether the integrity of the ocular surface epithelium in patients with AD is impaired. In a study of AD patients with blepharoconjunctivitis who were age matched with patients with seasonal or perennial allergic conjunctivitis and normals, the AD plus blepharocon-junctivitis patients showed significantly higher fluorescein uptake in the cornea and bulbar conjunctiva than the normals and patients with allergic conjunctivitis.[21]

Other abnormalities in AKC include epithelial pseudotubule formation and goblet cell hyperplasia,[22] increased basophil histamine release, eosinophilia, and elevated serum IgE. Conjunctivae from patients with AKC have a marked increase of CD3$^+$ lymphocytes, primarily CD4$^+$ phenotype in the substantia propria. In addition, the conjunctivae express increased IL-4 and IL-5. These cells also express the TCR-α/β phenotype. In addition, there is an increase in CD1$^+$ Langerhans cells noted in the epithelium and the substantia propria. As expected in patients with AD, the serum IgE is commonly elevated in patients with AKC, but correlates poorly with the severity of disease.[23] The highest levels of serum IgE seem to be found in those patients with atopic cataracts compared with normals.[24] Tears from AKC patients may have IgE, eosinophils, and mononuclear cells with a paucity of basophils and mast cells. This is in contrast to patients with atopic blepharoconjunctivitis.

CLINICAL MANIFESTATIONS
Epidemiology and Concomitant Disorders

It is commonly accepted that atopy affects 5% to 20% of the general population. The prevalence of AD in children is as high as 20%, whereas AKC occurs in 20% to 40% of individuals with AD, although it is uncommon to find AKC as a sole manifestation of atopy.[25,26] AKC is associated a familial history for atopy, such as AD and asthma, and over 95% of AKC patients also have eczema and 87% have a history of asthma. The inverse, however (ie, the reported incidence of ocular involvement in patients with AD), reveals a range of 25% to 42%.[23,27–29] Although there have been a few case reports of patients diagnosed with AKC as the sole manifestation of their atopy, these patients had a long-standing history of chronic conjunctivitis with bilateral pannus formation. Further evaluation by an allergy specialist revealed that they all had features of a more systemic atopic disorder including AD and asthma.[30]

The symptoms of AKC commonly include itching, burning, and tearing, which are much more severe than in seasonal or perennial allergic conjunctivitis and tend to be present throughout the year. Seasonal exacerbations are reported in many patients, especially in the winter or summer months,[14] and with exposure to animal dander, dust, and certain foods. There seems to be a trend in AD patients having ocular involvement with increasing levels of IgE and specific IgE to foods, such as rice and wheat and allergic mediators.[16]

AKC most commonly involves the lower tarsal conjunctiva and when it involves the cornea, it can lead to blindness. Originally reported to flare with worsening dermatitis, there are reports that some patients' ocular involvement evolves independently of their dermatitis,[2] whereas other reports reflect a correlation with tear levels of eosinophil cationic protein.[31]

AKC presents in the late teens and early twenties and may persist until the fourth and fifth decades of life.[14] The disorder only occasionally presents before the late teenage years. When AKC is noted to start earlier, however, it is characterized by greater ocular surface epithelial damage.[32] Conversely, severe AKC associated with complications, such as blepharoconjunctivitis, cataract, corneal disease, and ocular herpes simplex, occurs primarily in older patients with a peak incidence occurring in the 30- to 50-year-old age group.[27,33,34]

Ocular complications are seen in over a third of patients with AD, ranging from 31% to 43%[27] to 56%.[35] Ocular involvement was reported in 41 of 128 patients with AD: 13 had severe conjunctivitis and three had severe keratitis.[29] Similarly, in another study, 85 out of 200 patients with AD were reported to have ocular involvement including blepharoconjunctivitis, cataract, corneal scarring, pannus formation, keratoconus, and ocular herpes simplex.[27] Severe active AD treated in an ophthalmologic service revealed predominant clinical features of eyelid eczema (66%), AKC, superficial punctate keratopathy (68%), and decreased tear function tests (56%).[36]

In addition to the cutaneous manifestations of AD, the periorbital skin and cheeks are commonly involved in AKC with eczematoid changes including erythema and thick and dry scales.[37] Dennie-Morgan lines involving the skin of the eyelid result in a single or double infraorbital crease secondary to edema or thickening. As with seasonal and perennial allergic conjunctivitis, allergic shiners are common. The absence of the lateral eyebrow is present in many older patients (de Hertoghe sign) and may be caused by the extensive chronic eye rubbing or some form of autonomic dysfunction.[38,39] Signs include bilateral involvement of the conjunctiva (primarily lower tarsal) in the form of fine papillary hypertrophy of conjunctiva, chemosis, limbal hyperemia, and limbal gelatinous hyperplasia.

In a study reported in 1990 that involved a 9-year retrospective review of 45 patients seen at a large referral center the severity of ocular disease was quite pronounced with subepithelial fibrosis (N = 26), symblepharon or fornix foreshortening (N = 13), and severe keratopathy (N = 34), which included neovascularization in 17 patients. Persistent epithelial defect was another major complication, occurring in 21 eyes and causing severe loss of vision.[14] The description of the more severe forms of AKC is similar to cicatrizing conjunctivitis or cicatricial pemphigoid with subepithelial fibrosis, fornix shortening, and symblepharon formation.[23] Bilateral involvement with abundant mucoid discharge is the rule. Secondary staphylococcal blepharitis is common, caused by the eyelids becoming indurated and macerated. AKC is a chronic inflammatory allergic disease associated with conjunctival and corneal complications that include superficial punctate keratitis, macroerosions, corneal ulceration, plaque formation, corneal neovascularization, and lipid infiltration. The bulbar conjunctiva is commonly injected and chemotic. The corneal epithelium reveals punctate staining with fluorescein and limbal infiltration, Horner points, or Trantas dots. It is the corneal scarring and neovascularization, however, that may result in blindness. Keratoconus occurs in a small percentage (1.5%–16%) of patients with AD[40,41]; conversely, AD was reported to occur in 16% of patients with keratoconus.[40] In a recent study of AD, eyelid eczema (66%), AKC, and superficial punctate keratopathy (68%) were the dominant ocular diseases.

COMPLICATIONS

Blepharitis involving predominantly the skin and lashes tends to be staphylococcal or seborrheic in nature, whereas involvement of the meibomian glands may be either seborrheic; obstructive; or a combination (mixed). The pathophysiology of blepharitis is a complex interaction of various factors, including abnormal lid-margin secretions, microbial organisms, and abnormalities of the tear film. Blepharitis can present with a range of signs and symptoms, and is associated with various dermatologic conditions, including seborrheic dermatitis, rosacea, and eczema. The mainstay of treatment is an eyelid hygiene regimen, which needs to be continued long-term. Topical antibiotics are used to reduce the bacterial load. Topical corticosteroid preparations may be helpful in patients with marked inflammation.[42]

Individuals with AD have frequent colonization and infection with S aureus. AD patients have problems with synthesizing defensin proteins (eg, human β-defensin-3) associated with the rapid elimination of S aureus.[43] AKC patients generate increased α-defensin levels in tears.[44] It is unclear whether there is a subset of AKC patients with similar problems to those found in the skin that may lead to secondary staphylococcal blepharoconjunctivitis. Other specific ocular complications of AD include cataracts, blepharitis, keratoconus, iritis, and retinal detachment.

Cataracts as an ocular complication of AD were reported in 1914.[45,46] AKC occurs in 8% to 12% of patients with the severe form of AD, but especially in young adults approximately 10 years after the onset of the AD.[41,47–51] It is in this more severe population that cataracts are observed.[50] A unique feature of AKC cataracts is that they predominantly involve the anterior portion of the lens and may evolve rapidly into complete opacification within 6 months. Patients with AD may also develop posterior or nuclear type cataracts that may not be distinguishable from steroid-induced cataracts.[27,48,52–57] The use of oral or prolonged topical corticosteroid therapy may increase progression of atopic cataract formation or may cause the classical homogenous posterior cataract. There is a suggestion that high levels of IgE[16] or the rapid rise of IgE levels may portend the development of atopic cataracts.[24] In patients diagnosed with an atopic cataract on the first visit, IgE levels were approximately 25,000 IU/mL, whereas those who did not have cataracts had IgE levels of approximately 4000 IU/mL that increased to 13,000 IU/mL at the time of cataract development.[24] More recently, the 56T allele in the IFNGR1 promoter resulted in higher IFN-γ receptor 1 transcriptional activity and seems to be a genetic risk factor for atopic cataracts.[58] Although filaggrin has been associated with more severe forms of AD, hyperlinear palms, and keratosis pilaris, it has not been specifically evaluated for the development of AKC.[59,60]

Keratoconus is a progressive noninflammatory corneal ectasia that occurs in a small percentage of patients with AD. There is an association between positive allergy skin tests and keratoconus.[61] AD is less common in patients with unilateral keratoconus and keratoconus occurs more frequently on the side of the dominant hand. Although keratoconus patients with and without atopy did not differ significantly with regard to gender, age of onset, or rate of keratoplasty, it has been noted that patients with very high IgE levels were more prone to graft rejection.[61]

Postkeratoplasty atopic sclerokeratitis is a potentially severe complication in atopic patients undergoing keratoplasty. In the evaluation of postsurgical complications of patients (N = 247 keratoconus eyes) undergoing keratoplasty, 14% had a history of AD, of which six eyes of five patients (2.4%) developed postkeratoplasty atopic sclerokeratitis. The mean age of postkeratoplasty atopic sclerokeratitis patients was 29 years with the mean onset of postkeratoplasty atopic sclerokeratitis being 26 days. Preoperative atopic blepharitis and corneal neovascularization were identified as risk factors for postkeratoplasty atopic sclerokeratitis.[62] Inversely, eczema was reported to occur in 16% of patients with keratoconus.[40]

Retinal detachment seems to be increased in patients with AKC and in AD.[63–66] Additional complications of AKC including blepharoconjunctivitis, cataract, corneal disease, and ocular herpes simplex are commonly associated with older patients and have been reported to be as high as 42.5%.[25,33,67] Herpes simplex keratitis is often bilateral with high recurrence rates that are more severe. Many patients may develop secondary staphylococcal blepharitis. It seems that AKC patients have a higher incidence of bacterial superinfections, especially with staphylococcus.[1,68] In a recent study, S aureus was isolated from 67% of the AD patients, and finding any type of bacteria was isolated from 86% of the patients was significantly higher than those of nonatopic control participants (6% S aureus and 25% any bacteria). No significant relationship between the frequency distribution of bacteria and the grade of atopy or associated ocular diseases was noted, however, in this small population of AD patients (N = 36).[69]

AKC with significant epithelial disease also demonstrates decreased corneal sensitivity and tear film break-up times, compared with patients with insignificant epithelial disease and controls (P<.01).[70]

The dermal and conjunctival irritation associated with staphylococcal colonization was postulated as early as 1937, suggesting that the inflammatory response was induced by a "dermonecrotic factor." It was histologically noted that no lymph follicles or eosinophils were present with several types of keratitis and corneal involvement. Epithelial keratitis can be caused by "toxic mechanisms."[71–73] AKC patients have similar findings to those hypothesized from staphylococcal colonization with various degrees of ocular surface alterations that include superficial punctate keratitis, macroerosions, corneal ulceration, plaque formation, corneal neovascularization, and lipid infiltration. These lesions mimic some of the pathologic features seen in asthma, such as Creola bodies, desquamated bronchial linings that have been associated with the deposition of major basic protein. Early studies demonstrated a correlation of tear eosinophil cationic protein levels with severity of ocular disease.[31] Finding the heavily infiltrated mucosal surface of AKC patients with various inflammatory mediators and cells associated with atopy, such as mast cells, eosinophils, and lymphocytes, has led many to investigate the direct effect of eosinophilic mediators, such as tear eosinophilic cationic protein or major basic protein. Studies have shown their presence, their involvement in animal models, and a direct correlation with such treatments as mitomycin C aided papillary resection provided a dramatic decrease in ocular surface inflammation as evidenced by decrease in the number of inflammatory cells and tear eosinophil cationic protein levels with a rapid improvement of clinical corneal and conjunctival findings.[74] Eosinophils are uncommon in seasonal and perennial forms of allergic conjunctivitis, but are found in AKC. Recent studies show that the incidence of concurrent infection (mainly bacterial infections caused by S aureus) strongly correlated with the percent of eosinophilic cells. Concurrent bacterial infection was identified in 26 of 26 cases of the subgroup with the highest percent of eosinophilic cells.[75] In addition, tear film dysfunction seems to coexist with AKC as demonstrated by tear break-up time values of less than 10 seconds in 62% of the eyes and C 1, 2, and 4 mRNA expression.[70,76] Impression cytology samples from eyes with corneal ulcers showed significant squamous metaplasia and reduction in goblet cell density compared with eyes without ulcers and eyes of control subjects. Specimens from eyes with corneal ulcers showed periodic acid–Schiff positive mucin pickup and did not stain positive for MUC5AC. MUC5AC mRNA expression was significantly lower in eyes with corneal ulcers compared with eyes without ulcers and eyes of control subjects. MUC5AC mRNA expression was also significantly lower in eyes with AKC suggesting that ocular surface inflammation in patients with AKC has tear film instability and decreased conjunctival mucins in the tear fluid layer that may be important in the pathogenesis of noninfectious corneal shield ulcers in atopic ocular surface disease.[70,76–78]

NASAL-OCULAR LINKS IN AKC

Various forms of chronic ocular allergy exist, but there are limited studies to demonstrate the significance of the relationship between the chronic forms of allergic keratoconjunctivitis (atopic and vernal) and allergic rhinitis. In a recent allergen nasal challenge, ocular symptoms were collected in addition to the nasal symptoms from atopic (N = 15) showing positive history and skin tests, but responding insufficiently to the local ophthalmologic therapy with a control population of allergic rhinitis (N = 11) who did not have a history of ocular disease. It is interesting to note that out of 71 allergen nasal challenges 51 positive nasal responses were noted in 24 patients (P<.01), and 43 (<80%) of the nasal challenges were accompanied by significant ocular response (P<.01). No ocular responses were measured during the 26 phosphate buffered saline control nasal challenges (P>.05) or during 11 repeated nasal provocations in control subjects (P>.2). The results provide additional evidence for possible involvement of nasal allergy in some of the chronic forms of ocular allergy that commonly involve more than just mast cells in the involvement of the cornea (ie, keratoconjunctivitis).[79] Twenty years earlier the same author had proposed a nasal-ocular linkage.[80]

TREATMENT

Medical treatments for AKC have included mast cell stabilizing agents, such as cromolyn,[81] Iodoxamide,[82,83] N-acetylaspartylglutamic acid,[83] anti-IgE,[84] plasmapheresis,[85] and newer immunomodulatory agents for the treatment of severe AKC.[86–90] The use of cyclosporine and tacrolimus has proved effective in the treatment of both AD and AKC in a small number of patients.[91,92] A topical cyclosporin formula has also been shown to improve subjective and objective symptoms and signs of AKC.[93,94] In the latter study, 30% of steroid users were able to discontinue topical steroids,[94] whereas in another study of 18 AKC patients the use of a lower concentration of a topical cyclosporin A 0.05% ointment as a steroid-sparing agent was not found to be better than placebo.[95]

Various reports have described the use of topical calcineurin inhibitors in the treatment of periocular AD.[91,96] Topical tacrolimus 0.1% ointment reduced signs and symptoms of eyelid eczema.[97] There are two studies listed focusing on the treatment of AKC using topical cyclosporine in a solution versus the presently approved suspension for tear film dysfunction (http://clinicaltrials.gov/ct2/show/NCT00884585?term= atopic+keratoconjunctivitis&rank=2. Accessed December 25, 2009).[98,99] In the more severe forms, however, systemic treatment with calcineurin inhibitors or daclizumab may be required.[96]

Contact lenses have also been used in some patients with AKC. Specifically, rigid gas-permeable scleral contact lenses were used in the treatment and visual rehabilitation of patients with advanced AKC and demonstrated improved vision with their use for more than 18 months.[100,101]

SUMMARY

AD is one of the chronic diseases seen by allergist-immunologists that have both dermatologic and ocular manifestations. The occurrence of ocular disease is often proportionately higher than that of dermatologic disease. Even if the skin abnormalities seem well controlled, these patients require ophthalmic evaluation. Optimal management requires a team approach that includes the primary care physician, allergist, and ophthalmologist. AKC in AD patients is characterized by acute exacerbations and requires maintenance therapy for long-term control. Exacerbations need aggressive treatment to limit ocular signs and symptoms and to reduce ocular inflammation that can lead to permanent visual loss. Hygiene cannot be overemphasized because colonization with S aureus may be associated with the local release of superantigenic exotoxins generating a form of toxic shock syndrome of the eye that over time leads to more severe complications of AKC. Topical corticosteroid use, although at times needed, should be minimized to decrease the potential adverse effect on the eye (glaucoma and cataracts). Future studies will continue to emphasize the use of steroid-sparing, immunomodulating agents that have the potential to provide long-lasting anti-inflammatory control with a more favorable side-effect profile. Overall, AKC is more common than previously appreciated, because it was primarily recognized only in the more severe forms, whereas milder forms are seen by practicing allergist-immunologists and these patients need to be identified and treated earlier to prevent disabling visual abnormalities.

REFERENCES

1. Hogan MJ. Atopic keratoconjunctivitis. Trans Am Acad Ophthalmol Otolaryngol 1952;50:265–81 (88th Meet).
2. Hogan MJ. Atopic keratoconjunctivitis. Am J Ophthalmol 1953;36(7:1):937–47.
3. Bielory L. Ocular allergy overview. Immunol Allergy Clin North Am 2008;28(1): 1–23.
4. Bielory L, Friedlaender MH. Allergic conjunctivitis. Immunol Allergy Clin North Am 2008;28(1):43–58.
5. Leonardi A, De Dominicis C, Motterle L. Immunopathogenesis of ocular allergy: a schematic approach to different clinical entities. Curr Opin Allergy Clin Immunol 2007;7(5):429–35.
6. Leonardi A, Fregona IA, Plebani M, et al. Th1- and Th2-type cytokines in chronic ocular allergy. Graefes Arch Clin Exp Ophthalmol 2006;244(10):1240–5.
7. Metz DP, Hingorani M, Calder VL, et al. T-cell cytokines in chronic allergic eye disease. J Allergy Clin Immunol 1997;100(6 Pt 1):817–24.
8. Nivenius E, Montan PG, Chryssanthou E, et al. No apparent association between periocular and ocular microcolonization and the degree of inflammation in patients with atopic keratoconjunctivitis. Clin Exp Allergy 2004;34(5):725–30.
9. Uchio E, Ono SY, Ikezawa Z, et al. Tear levels of interferon-gamma, interleukin (IL)-2, IL-4 and IL-5 in patients with vernal keratoconjunctivitis, atopic keratoconjunctivitis and allergic conjunctivitis. Clin Exp Allergy 2000;30:103–9.
10. Matsuura N, Uchio E, Nakazawa M, et al. Predominance of infiltrating IL-4-producing T cells in conjunctiva of patients with allergic conjunctival disease. Curr Eye Res 2004;29(4–5):235–43.
11. Avunduk AM, Avunduk MC, Dayanir V, et al. Further studies on the immunopathology of atopic keratoconjunctivitis using flow cytometry. Exp Eye Res 1997; 65:803–8.
12. Yoshida A, Imayama S, Sugai S, et al. Increased number of IgE positive Langerhans cells in the conjunctiva of patients with atopic dermatitis. Br J Ophthalmol 1997;81(5):402–6.
13. Matsuda A, Okayama Y, Ebihara N, et al. Hyperexpression of the high-affinity IgE receptor-beta chain in chronic allergic keratoconjunctivitis. Invest Ophthalmol Vis Sci 2009;50(6):2871–7.
14. Foster CS, Calonge M. Atopic keratoconjunctivitis. Ophthalmology 1990;97(8): 992–1000.
15. Tabbara KF, Nassar A, Ahmed SO, et al. Acquisition of vernal and atopic keratoconjunctivitis after bone marrow transplantation. Am J Ophthalmol 2008; 146(3):462–5.
16. Uchio E, Miyakawa K, Ikezawa Z, et al. Systemic and local immunological features of atopic dermatitis patients with ocular complications. Br J Ophthalmol 1998;82(1):82–7.

17. Taniguchi H, Ohki O, Yokozeki H, et al. Cataract and retinal detachment in patients with severe atopic dermatitis who were withdrawn from the use of topical corticosteroid. J Dermatol 1999;26(10):658–65.

18. Toshitani A, Imayama S, Shimozono Y, et al. Reduced amount of secretory component of IgA secretion in tears of patients with atopic dermatitis. J Dermatol Sci 1999;19(2):134–8.

19. Cook EB, Stahl JL, Esnault S, et al. Toll-like receptor 2 expression on human conjunctival epithelial cells: a pathway for Staphylococcus aureus involvement in chronic ocular proinflammatory responses. Ann Allergy Asthma Immunol 2005;94(4):486–97.

20. Chung SH, Nam KH, Kweon MN. Staphylococcus aureus accelerates an experimental allergic conjunctivitis by Toll-like receptor 2-dependent manner. Clin Immunol 2009;131(1):170–7.

21. Yokoi K, Yokoi N, Kinoshita S. Impairment of ocular surface epithelium barrier function in patients with atopic dermatitis. Br J Ophthalmol 1998;82(7): 797–800.

22. Foster CS, Rice BA, Dutt JE. Immunopathology of atopic keratoconjunctivitis. Ophthalmology 1991;98(8):1190–6.

23. Tuft SJ, Kemeny DM, Dart JK, et al. Clinical features of atopic keratoconjunctivitis. Ophthalmology 1991;98(2):150–8.

24. Sasabe T, Suwa Y, Kawamura T, et al. [Cataracts occur in patients with atopic dermatitis when the serum IgE increases]. Nippon Ganka Gakkai Zasshi 1997;101(5):389–92 [in Japanese].

25. Bielory L. Allergic and immunologic disorders of the eye. Part II: ocular allergy. J Allergy Clin Immunol 2000;106(6):1019–32.

26. Bielory L. Allergic and immunologic disorders of the eye. Part I: immunology of the eye. J Allergy Clin Immunol 2000;106(5):805–16.

27. Garrity JA, Liesegang TJ. Ocular complications of atopic dermatitis. Can J Ophthalmol 1984;19(1):21–4.

28. Karel I, Myska V, Kvicalova E. [Eye changes in atopic dermatitis]. Cesk Oftalmol 1963;19:130–8 [in Czech].

29. Karel I, Myska V, Kvicalova E. Ophthalmological changes in atopic dermatitis. Acta Derm Venereol 1965;45(5):381–6.

30. Akova YA, Jabbur NS, Neumann R, et al. Atypical ocular atopy. Ophthalmology 1993;100(9):1367–71.

31. Montan PG, van Hage-Hamsten M. Eosinophil cationic protein in tears in allergic conjunctivitis. Br J Ophthalmol 1996;80(6):556–60.

32. Onguchi T, Dogru M, Okada N, et al. The impact of the onset time of atopic keratoconjunctivitis on the tear function and ocular surface findings. Am J Ophthalmol 2006;141(3):569–71.

33. Oshinskie L, Haine C. Atopic dermatitis and its ophthalmic complications. J Am Optom Assoc 1982;53(11):889–94.

34. Rich LF, Hanifin JM. Ocular complications of atopic dermatitis and other eczemas. Int Ophthalmol Clin 1985;25(1):61–76.

35. Ohmachi N, Sasabe T, Kojima M, et al. [Eye complications in atopic dermatitis]. Arerugi 1994;43(7):796–9 [in Japanese].

36. Dogru M, Nakagawa N, Tetsumoto K, et al. Ocular surface disease in atopic dermatitis. Jpn J Ophthalmol 1999;43(1):53–7.

37. Peralejo B, Beltrani V, Bielory L. Dermatologic and allergic conditions of the eyelid. Immunol Allergy Clin North Am 2008;28(1):137–68.

38. Nagaraja, Kanwar AJ, Dhar S, et al. Frequency and significance of minor clinical features in various age-related subgroups of atopic dermatitis in children. Pediatr Dermatol 1996;13(1):10–3.
39. Polemann G, Peltzer L. [The eye brow sign of Hertoghe, a symptom of function of the autonomic nervous system]. Medizinische 1952;31(25):856–60.
40. Copeman PW. Eczema and keratoconus. Br Med J 1965;5468:977–9.
41. Amemiya T, Matsuda H, Uehara M. Ocular findings in atopic dermatitis with special reference to the clinical features of atopic cataract. Ophthalmologica 1980;180(3):129–32.
42. Jackson WB. Blepharitis: current strategies for diagnosis and management. Can J Ophthalmol 2008;43(2):170–9.
43. Kisich KO, Carspecken CW, Fiéve S, et al. Defective killing of Staphylococcus aureus in atopic dermatitis is associated with reduced mobilization of human beta-defensin-3. J Allergy Clin Immunol 2008;122(1):62–8.
44. Hida RY, Ohashi Y, Takano Y, et al. Elevated levels of human alpha-defensin in tears of patients with allergic conjunctival disease complicated by corneal lesions: detection by SELDI ProteinChip system and quantification. Curr Eye Res 2005;30(9):723–30.
45. Beetham W. Atopic cataracts. Arch Ophtalmol 1940;24:21–37.
46. Brunsting LA, Reed WB, Bair HL. Occurrence of cataracts and keratoconus with atopic dermatitis. AMA Arch Derm 1955;72(3):237–41.
47. Kornerup T, Lodin A. Ocular changes in 100 cases of Besnier's prurigo (atopic dermatitis). Acta Ophthalmol (Copenh) 1959;37:508–21.
48. Uehara M, Sato T. Atopic cataract induced by severe allergic contact dermatitis on the face. Dermatologica 1986;172(1):54–7.
49. Uehara M, Amemiya T, Arai M. Atopic cataracts in a Japanese population. With special reference to factors possibly relevant to cataract formation. Dermatologica 1985;170(4):180–4.
50. Ibarra-Duran MG, Mena-Cedillos CA, Rodriguez-Almaraz M. [Cataracts and atopic dermatitis in children. A study of 68 patients]. Bol Med Hosp Infant Mex 1992;49(12):851–5 [in Spanish].
51. Ewing CI, Roper HP, David TJ, et al. Death from eczema herpeticum in a child with severe eczema, mental retardation and cataracts. J R Soc Med 1989;82(3):169–70.
52. Urban RC Jr, Cotlier E. Corticosteroid-induced cataracts. Surv Ophthalmol 1986;31(2):102–10.
53. Toogood JH, Markov AE, Baskerville J, et al. Association of ocular cataracts with inhaled and oral steroid therapy during long-term treatment of asthma. J Allergy Clin Immunol 1993;91(2):571–9.
54. Tatham A. Atopic dermatitis, cutaneous steroids and cataracts in children: two case reports. J Med Case Reports 2008;2:124.
55. Ferguson JG Jr, Marshall C. Atopic dermatitis and cataracts. Va Med 1977;104(4):258–60.
56. Castrow FF II. Atopic cataracts versus steroid cataracts. J Am Acad Dermatol 1981;5(1):64–6.
57. Bielory L. Ocular toxicity of systemic asthma and allergy treatments. Curr Allergy Asthma Rep 2006;6(4):299–305.
58. Matsuda A, Ebihara N, Kumagai N, et al. Genetic polymorphisms in the promoter of the interferon gamma receptor 1 gene are associated with atopic cataracts. Invest Ophthalmol Vis Sci 2007;48(2):583–9.

59. Bremmer SF, Hanifin JM, Simpson EL. Clinical detection of ichthyosis vulgaris in an atopic dermatitis clinic: implications for allergic respiratory disease and prognosis. J Am Acad Dermatol 2008;59(1):72–8.

60. Komine M. Analysis of the mechanism for the development of allergic skin inflammation and the application for its treatment: keratinocytes in atopic dermatitis—their pathogenic involvement. J Pharmacol Sci 2009;110(3): 260–4.

61. Harrison RJ, Klouda PT, Easty DL, et al. Association between keratoconus and atopy. Br J Ophthalmol 1989;73(10):816–22.

62. Tomita M, Shimmura S, Tsubota K, et al. Postkeratoplasty atopic sclerokeratitis in keratoconus patients. Ophthalmology 2008;115(5):851–6.

63. Coles RS, Laval J. Retinal detachments occurring in cataract associated with neurodermatitis. AMA Arch Opthalmol 1952;48(1):30–9.

64. Hurlbut WB, Domonkos AN. Cataract and retinal detachment associated with atopic dermatitis. AMA Arch Opthalmol 1954;52(6):852–7.

65. Ingram RM. Retinal detachment associated with atopic dermatitis and cataract. Br J Ophthalmol 1965;49:96–7.

66. Katsushima H, Miyazaki I, Sekine N, et al. [Incidence of cataract and retinal detachment associated with atopic dermatitis]. Nippon Ganka Gakkai Zasshi 1994;98(5):495–500 [in Japanese].

67. Easty D, Entwistle C, Funk A, et al. Herpes simplex keratitis and keratoconus in the atopic patient. A clinical and immunological study. Trans Ophthalmol Soc U K 1975;95(2):267–76.

68. Tuft SJ, Ramakrishnan M, Seal DV, et al. Role of *Staphylococcus aureus* in chronic allergic conjunctivitis. Ophthalmology 1992;99(2):180–4.

69. Nakata K, Inoue Y, Harada J, et al. A high incidence of *Staphylococcus aureus* colonization in the external eyes of patients with atopic dermatitis. Ophthalmology 2000;107(12):2167–71.

70. Dogru M, Okada N, Asano-Kato N, et al. Alterations of the ocular surface epithelial mucins 1, 2, 4 and the tear functions in patients with atopic keratoconjunctivitis. Clin Exp Allergy 2006;36(12):1556–65.

71. Tetz MR, Klein U, Volcker HE. [*Staphylococcus*-associated blepharokeratoconjunctivitis. Clinical findings, pathogenesis and therapy]. Ophthalmologe 1997; 94(3):186–90 [in German].

72. Cvenkel B, Globocnik M. Conjunctival scrapings and impression cytology in chronic conjunctivitis. Correlation with microbiology. Eur J Ophthalmol 1997; 7(1):19–23.

73. Kerr N, Stern GA. Bacterial keratitis associated with vernal keratoconjunctivitis. Cornea 1992;11(4):355–9.

74. Tanaka M, Dogru M, Takano Y, et al. Quantitative evaluation of the early changes in ocular surface inflammation following MMC-aided papillary resection in severe allergic patients with corneal complications. Cornea 2006;25(3): 281–5.

75. Forte R, Cennamo G, Del Prete S, et al. Allergic conjunctivitis and latent infections. Cornea 2009;28(8):839–42.

76. Dogru M, Asano-Kato N, Tanaka M, et al. Ocular surface and MUC5AC alterations in atopic patients with corneal shield ulcers. Curr Eye Res 2005;30(10): 897–908.

77. Dogru M, Okada N, Asano-Kato N, et al. Atopic ocular surface disease: implications on tear function and ocular surface mucins. Cornea 2005;24(Suppl 8): S18–23.

78. Dogru M, Ozmen A, Ertürk H, et al. Changes in tear function and the ocular surface after topical olopatadine treatment for allergic conjunctivitis: an open-label study. Clin Ther 2002;24(8):1309–21.
79. Pelikan Z. The possible involvement of nasal allergy in allergic keratoconjunctivitis. Eye 2008;23(8):1653–60.
80. Pelikan Z. [Allergic conjunctivitis; primary and secondary role of the allergic reaction in the nose]. Ned Tijdschr Geneeskd 1988;132(13):561–3 [in Dutch].
81. Jay JL. Clinical features and diagnosis of adult atopic keratoconjunctivitis and the effect of treatment with sodium cromoglycate. Br J Ophthalmol 1981; 65(5):335–40.
82. Giuri S, Munteanu GH. [An efficacy study of lodoxamide treatment in allergic eye lesions]. Oftalmologia 2000;50(1):68–76 [in Romanian].
83. Denis D, Bloch-Michel E, Verin P, et al. Treatment of common ocular allergic disorders; a comparison of lodoxamide and NAAGA. Br J Ophthalmol 1998; 82(10):1135–8.
84. Williams PB, Sheppard JD Jr. Omalizumab: a future innovation for treatment of severe ocular allergy? Expert Opin Biol Ther 2005;5(12):1603–9.
85. Aswad MI, Tauber J, Baum J. Plasmapheresis treatment in patients with severe atopic keratoconjunctivitis. Ophthalmology 1988;95(4):444–7.
86. Scheinfeld N. A review of deferasirox, bortezomib, dasatinib, and cyclosporine eye drops: possible uses and known side effects in cutaneous medicine. J Drugs Dermatol 2007;6(3):352–5.
87. Ono SJ, Abelson MB. Allergic conjunctivitis: update on pathophysiology and prospects for future treatment. J Allergy Clin Immunol 2005;115(1):118–22.
88. Leonardi A. Emerging drugs for ocular allergy. Expert Opin Emerg Drugs 2005; 10(3):505–20.
89. Bielory L, Kempuraj D, Theoharides T. Topical immunopharmacology of ocular allergies. Curr Opin Allergy Clin Immunol 2002;2(5):435–45.
90. Origlieri C, Bielory L. Emerging drugs for conjunctivitis. Expert Opin Emerg Drugs 2009;14(3):523–36.
91. Zribi H, Descamps V, Hoang-Xuan T, et al. Dramatic improvement of atopic keratoconjunctivitis after topical treatment with tacrolimus ointment restricted to the eyelids. J Eur Acad Dermatol Venereol 2009;23(4):489–90.
92. Stumpf T, Luqmani N, Sumich P, et al. Systemic tacrolimus in the treatment of severe atopic keratoconjunctivitis. Cornea 2006;25(10):1147–9.
93. Ozcan AA, Ersoz TR, Dulger E. Management of severe allergic conjunctivitis with topical cyclosporin a 0.05% eyedrops. Cornea 2007;26(9):1035–8.
94. Ebihara N, Ohashi Y, Uchio E, et al. A large prospective observational study of novel cyclosporine 0.1% aqueous ophthalmic solution in the treatment of severe allergic conjunctivitis. J Ocul Pharmacol Ther 2009;25(4):365–72.
95. Daniell M, Constantinou M, Vu HT, et al. Randomised controlled trial of topical ciclosporin A in steroid dependent allergic conjunctivitis. Br J Ophthalmol 2006;90(4):461–4.
96. Anzaar F, Gallagher MJ, Bhat P, et al. Use of systemic T-lymphocyte signal transduction inhibitors in the treatment of atopic keratoconjunctivitis. Cornea 2008; 27(8):884–8.
97. Nivenius E, van der Ploeg I, Jung K, et al. Tacrolimus ointment vs steroid ointment for eyelid dermatitis in patients with atopic keratoconjunctivitis. Eye 2007;21(7):968–75.
98. Bielory L. Ocular allergy and dry eye syndrome. Curr Opin Allergy Clin Immunol 2004;4(5):421–4.

99. Bielory L. Differential diagnoses of conjunctivitis for clinical allergist-immunologists. Ann Allergy Asthma Immunol 2007;98(2):105–14 [quiz: 114–7, 152].
100. Margolis R, Thakrar V, Perez VL. Role of rigid gas-permeable scleral contact lenses in the management of advanced atopic keratoconjunctivitis. Cornea 2007;26(9):1032–4.
101. Lemp MA, Bielory L. Contact lenses and associated anterior segment disorders: dry eye disease, blepharitis, and allergy. Immunol Allergy Clin North Am 2008; 28(1):105–17.

The Role of Contact Allergy in Atopic Dermatitis

Luz S. Fonacier, MD[a,b],*, Marcella R. Aquino, MD[a,c]

KEYWORDS

• Allergic contact dermatitis • Atopic dermatitis • Patch testing

BACKGROUND AND PATHOGENESIS

Atopic dermatitis (AD) causes a significant economic and quality-of-life burden among the 15.2 million Americans who have this disease, according to estimates from the Society of Investigative Dermatology and American Academy of Dermatology study. Almost five times that number (72.4 million) suffer from contact dermatitis (CD).[1] A previously held belief was that patients with AD were less likely to have allergic contact dermatitis (ACD) than the general population because of the presence of decreased lymphocyte-mediated hypersensitivity.

AD was traditionally considered mostly an IgE-mediated disease (extrinsic AD) in which T cells with the skin-homing receptor cutaneous lymphocyte–associated antigen (CLA) produce Th2 cytokines after encountering allergens in lymph nodes.[2,3] These cytokines promote growth of eosinophils and switch to IgE immunoglobulin production with concomitant reduction in cell-mediated immunity.[2] However these CLA+ T cells also produce low levels of interferon (IFN)-γ (a Th1 cytokine) that inhibit Th2 function and chronic AD skin lesions have increased numbers of interleukin (IL)-5, granulocyte-macrophage colony-stimulating factor (GM-CSF), IL-12, and IFN-γ– expressing cells.[4]

Clinically, patients with AD display an increased rate of viral (herpes simplex, human papillomavirus, molluscum contagiosum) and chronic dermatophyte infections but less susceptibility to poison ivy and cutaneous anergy to allergens.[5–7] However, the

Funding Support: none.
[a] Department of Internal Medicine, State University of New York at Stony Brook, 100 Nicolls Road, Stony Brook, NY 11790, USA
[b] Section of Allergy, Division of Rheumatology, Allergy and Immunology, Department of Internal Medicine, Winthrop University Hospital, 120 Mineola Boulevard, Suite 410, Mineola, NY 11501, USA
[c] Division of Rheumatology, Allergy & Immunology, Winthrop University Hospital, 120 Mineola Boulevard, Suite 410, Mineola, NY 11501, USA
* Corresponding author. Section of Allergy, Division of Rheumatology, Allergy & Immunology, Winthrop University Hospital, 120 Mineola Boulevard, Suite 410, Mineola, NY 11501.
E-mail address: lfonacier@winthrop.org

Immunol Allergy Clin N Am 30 (2010) 337–350
doi:10.1016/j.iac.2010.06.001
0889-8561/10/$ – see front matter © 2010 Elsevier Inc. All rights reserved.

epidermal skin barrier dysfunction in patients with AD facilitates introduction of foreign antigens. Filaggrin functions to aggregate keratin filaments, leading to formation of the stratum corneum layer, and it's defect has been linked to *Ichthyosis vulgaris* and AD.[8] This impaired barrier function may represent a mechanism for sensitization to topical agents, allergens, and microbes in atopics by facilitating the penetration of contact allergens and irritants into the epidermis.[2,9] Two filaggrin mutations were screened in a European cross-sectional population that underwent patch testing (PT) with a standard panel of 25 allergens.[9] Results suggest that the filaggrin loss of function mutations represent a risk factor for contact sensitization to nickel, especially in combination with a history of adverse reactions to jewelry.[9] No association with sensitization to other common allergens was seen.

IL-31 is a cytokine produced mainly by activated CD4+ T cells through a heterodimeric receptor to activate Jak/STAT, PI3K/AKT, and MAPK pathways; in mice models, it produces a pruritic dermatitis closely resembling AD.[10–12] Recent studies using polymerase chain reaction (PCR) have shown IL-31 in skin biopsies of patients with AD,[13] implying that this cytokine contributes to the development of inflammation and pruritus. Neis and colleagues[12] analyzed RNA from skin biopsy specimens from patients with AD, ACD, and psoriasis and from healthy controls. They found statistically significant increased levels of IL-31 mRNA in patients with AD; these levels were also increased in 24 of 56 patients with ACD but in none of those with psoriasis (n = 60).[12]

Similarities and differences are seen in CD and AD. Irritant contact dermatitis (ICD) results from contact with agents that abrade, irritate, or traumatize the skin, such as detergents, solvents, alcohol, lotions, and extreme wetness, dryness, or temperature. This perturbation of the skin barrier may lead to disorganization of the lipid bilayers in the epidermis[14] and increase of cytokine production (IL-1α and -β, tumor necrosis factor [TNF]-α, and GM-CSF) in the epidermis,[15] which can lead to direct tissue damage and increase in transepidermal water loss. ICD is nonimmunologic and does not require prior sensitization. The inflammatory response is dose- and time-dependent.

ACD is recognized as the prototypic type IV cutaneous cell–mediated hypersensitivity reaction. The environmental allergens are haptens that bind to carrier proteins to form complete antigens before they can cause sensitization. The hapten in the epidermis activates keratinocytes to release inflammatory cytokines and chemokines (TNF-α, GM-CSF, IL-1β, IL-10, and macrophage inflammatory protein [MIP]-2), which activate Langerhans cells, other dendritic cells, and endothelial cells. In the afferent limb, the Langerhans cells then process the antigen while migrating to regional lymph nodes, where they present it to naive T cells and cause the activation of CD4+ and CD8+ hapten-specific T cells.[16]

On subsequent exposure of the skin to the allergen, the sensitized T cells that home in to the hapten-provoked skin site release their inflammatory mediators that contribute to epidermal spongiosis (eczema). Spongiosis is the hallmark of the epidermis in eczema, whether caused by CD or AD. It is characterized by the widening of intercellular spaces, and intercellular edema that may progress to the formation of intraepidermal vesicles.

EPIDEMIOLOGY

Numerous studies in the early 1990s advocated the need for PT in patients with AD, reporting a frequency of 40% of ACD in patients with AD (**Table 1**). A prospective study performed in 137 atopic children in France showed a contact sensitization of

43% among children tested.[17] The most common allergens were metals (nickel, 19.3%), fragrance and lanolin (4.4%), Balsam of Peru (2.6%), and neomycin and emollients (2.6%). The children were negative to corticosteroids as screened by budesonide and tixocortol pivalate and children older than 5 years had a greater risk of developing contact allergy.[17]

A recent study in Poland performed in atopic school children and teenagers with eczema similarly found that 49.4% of 229 children tested had a positive PT.[18] These children (96 of whom were age 7 years and 133 were 16 years) underwent PT with a 10-allergen panel of the most frequent contact sensitizers in Europe. The most common positive results were to nickel sulfate (30.2%), thimerosal (10.4%), cobalt chloride (8.3%), and fragrance mix I (7.3%). Among the 16-year-olds, contact allergy to nickel was four times higher in girls with pierced ears than in those without. The diagnosis of ACD was confirmed to be relevant in 36.5% of the 7-year-olds and 26.3% of the 16-year-olds.[18]

In a smaller series of 30 children with AD in India with mild to moderate eczema, PT results for a standard panel of 31 antigens were positive in a smaller proportion of patients with AD.[19] Seven patients (23%) had a positive PT reaction to a total of eight allergens, the most common being neomycin and gentamycin, and those who had positive reactions had a longer duration of AD.

A prospective study from Tunisia in children and adults (63 children, 26 adults) with AD according to Hanifin and Rajka[20] criteria evaluated PT using the European Standard series, and supplemented with special series and personal products when necessary. Results showed PT to be positive in 42.7% and clinically relevant in 38.2% of overall subjects; and to be positive in 50% of adults and 39.7% of children, with nickel being the most common allergen.[21] Severity of AD was evaluated using the SCORAD (Scoring Atopic Dermatitis) index, which showed that positive PT reactions were more frequently seen in patients with severe AD (60.9%) than in those with moderate and mild AD (37.5% and 30%, respectively). These results correlated with the duration or course of AD. The authors speculated that numerous and prolonged topical treatments increase the risk of CD, in contrast to previous reports of reduced sensitization in patients with severe dermatitis.[22] This study found that risk of a positive PT reaction was significantly ($P = .017$) correlated with duration of AD.[21]

Mailhol and colleagues[23] examined 641 pediatric patients with AD for positive response to PT using antiseptics, emollients, and corticosteroids. All patients were tested to bufexamac, chlorhexidine, hexamidine, sodium fusidate, budesonide, tixocortol pivalate, and personal emollient. Among the children, 40 (6.2%) had 45 positive PT reactions. The allergens were emollients (47.5%), chlorhexidine (42.5%), hexamidine (7.5%), tixocortol pivalate (2.5%), and bufexamac (2.5%). Similar to results reported by Giordano-Labadie and colleagues,[17] 3% were positive to their current emollient. Assessment of age, sex, age of onset of AD, presence of asthma, SCORAD score, and skin prick testing in these patients showed that the following risk factors were associated with sensitization to topical treatment products in AD: (1) significantly younger age (2.8 years vs 4.8 years; $P<.001$), with onset of AD before 6 months of age (75% vs 53.1%, odds ratio [OR], 2.6); (2) more severe AD with higher SCORAD (29 vs 21; $P = .006$); and (3) IgE sensitization (OR, 2.5; 95% CI, 1.1–5.9). Neither sex nor history of asthma was associated with risk of sensitization to topical AD treatment. This study shows that although the prevalence of CD to treatments for AD is low, it is not negligible, and ACD in AD should be suspected, especially to antiseptics and emollients, when treatment fails to control the AD.

In a retrospective review of 110 children in the United Kingdom, certain subsets of patients with AD yielded higher positive PT results: patients with eyelid dermatitis

Table 1
Literature review

Author	Criteria for AD	Allergens Patch Tested	Results	Relevance
Giordano-Labadie et al[17]	Hanifin and Rajka 70 M:67 F Mean age: 4.5 y 42.7% mild 47% moderate 10.3% severe	European standard Series, tixocortol pivalate, budesonide, and emollient	43%, positive PT (49/114 tests) Metals, 19.3% Fragrance, 4.4% Lanolin, 4.4% Neomycin, 2.6% Emollient, 2.6%	All positive, relevant; avoidance led to SS improvement
Czarnobilska et al[18]	Patients screened for eczema based on questionnaire 96 children, aged 7 years 133 children aged 16 years	10 common contact allergens	49.4%, positive PT (Allergen, 7-year-old/ 16-year-old) Nickel, 30.2%/23.3% Thimerosal, 10.4%/27.8% Cobalt chloride, 8.3%/10.5%	36.5% of 7-year-olds; 26.3% of 16 year olds
Sharma et al[19]	Hanifin and Rajka 22M:8F Age, 7–50 years AD: mild to moderate	Indian standard battery	23%, positive PT Neomycin, 3/7 Gentamycin, 2/7	Relevance of positive PT was not discussed
Belhadjali et al[21]	Hanifin and Rajka 63 children (mean age, 69 months) 26 adults (mean age, 34 years)	European standard Series, special series, and personal products	42.7%, positive PT Nickel, 24.7% Chrome, 7.9% Cobalt chloride, 7.9% Parabens, 4.5% More PT positive in severe AD	38.2%

Mailhol et al[23]	UK Working Party 641 children Median age, 3.4 years 48%M:52%F 43%, moderate to severe AD	Chlorhexidine, hexamidine, budesonide, tixocortol pivalate, bufexamac, sodium fusidate, and emollient	6%, positive PT Emollients, 47.5% Chlorhexidine, 42.5% Hexamidine, 7.5% Tixocortol pivalate, 2.5%	Past relevance for most allergens
Beattie et al[24]	114 children 48M:66F Median age, 11.5 years Retrospective	66 to European series 48 to British Contact Dermatitis Group Series	54%, positive PT Nickel, 20% Rubber, 10% Fragrance, 7.2%	Current, past or possibly relevant in 54%
Mortz et al[25]	Hanifin and Rajka 1146 children 526M:620F	TRUE test panels 1 and 2	15.2% positive PT F>M positive results that were SS Nickel, 8.6% Fragrance mix, 1.8% F>M positive for nickel	Past or present in 47.7%
Ingordo et al[26]	280 consecutive adult patients with eczema Hanifin and Rajka AD group, 113M:2F Mean age, 21.3 y Non-AD, 78M:9F Mean age, 24.8 y	GIRDCA standard series	44.3% in AD group 51.7% in non-AD group Nickel was most positive antigen in both groups	Definite ACD in AD group, 29.6% Definite ACD in non-AD group, 35.6%

Abbreviations: AD, atopic dermatitis; F, female; GIRDCA, Gruppo Italiano Ricerca Dermatiti da Contatto e Ambientali; M, male; Neo, neomycin; PT, patch testing; SS, statistically significant; TRUE, thin layer rapid use epicutaneous test.

(86%), hand dermatitis (71%), and vulval dermatitis (100%).[24] However, patients who had been referred for worsening of their AD had the lowest rate of relevant positive reactions (22%), along with children with foot or facial dermatitis. Again, nickel was the most common allergen (22%), followed by rubber, fragrance, cobalt, and lanolin. None of the 47 children who underwent PT to corticosteroids had a positive response.

A cohort study conducted in adolescents in Denmark sought to determine prevalence of AD, asthma, allergic rhinitis, and hand and CD among 1501 eighth-grade students using questionnaire, interview, examination, and PT.[25] The lifetime prevalence of AD was 21.3%, 6.9% for allergic asthma, 15.7% for allergic rhinitis, and 9.2% for hand eczema. Significantly more girls had positive PT reactions to nickel,[25] but no other differences based on sex were noted for the 20 of 24 allergens that yielded positive PT results. In this study, 37% of patients with ACD had a history of AD.

In a group of mostly young men recruited to the Italian army, 280 consecutive adult patients with eczema underwent PT[26] with a standard series, with clinical relevance determined for all positive responses. These patients were divided into an atopic group and nonatopic group based on whether Hanifin and Rajka[20] criteria were fulfilled. PT showed no differences in sensitization, asserting at least the same incidence of ACD between atopic and nonatopic patients, with nickel, cobalt, and potassium dichromate as the most common allergens.[26]

COMMON AREAS OF INVOLVEMENT IN CD AND AD
Eyelids

Among patients with AD, 25% may have chronic eyelid dermatitis. However, dermatitis of the eyelid is most often caused by ACD (55%–63.5%). ICD accounts for 15% of eyelid dermatitis, AD accounts for less than 10%, and approximately 4% is attributed to seborrheic dermatitis.[27] Data collected by the North American Contact Dermatitis Group (NACDG) showed that in 193 (72%) of 268 patients with only eyelid dermatitis, gold was the most common allergen with a positive patch test. Fragrances, preservatives, nickel, thiuram, cocamidopropyl betaine and amidoamine (shampoos), and tosylamide formaldehyde resins (nail polish) were other allergens to consider in the evaluation of eyelid dermatitis.[28] In patients with mixed facial and eyelid dermatitis, nickel, Kathon, and fragrance were the most frequently positive on PT (**Fig. 1**).[29,30]

Lips

Lesions in the perioral region could be from lip licking, ACD, or AD. Among patients diagnosed by the NACDG with allergic cheilitis, 37% had at least 1 of the atopic triad.[31] Perioral dermatitis presents as small erythematous papules, vesicles, or tiny pustules and is most common in young women, but also occurs in prepubertal children of either sex. The causes are unknown, although topical glucocorticoid use seems to be a precipitating or exacerbating factor in some patients. Other proposed causative factors include contact allergy (eg, fluorinated toothpastes), occlusive moisturizers, and inhaled or systemic glucocorticoids.

Hands

The prevalence of hand eczema is two- to tenfold higher in patients with AD than in those without, and 16% have nail dystrophy. The increasing prevalence of hand involvement with advancing age is probably from repeated wetting and occupational insults, along with coexisting irritant dermatitis. Certain morphologic features can help distinguish the different contributing factors to hand eczema. Involvement of the dorsal hand and finger combined with volar wrist suggest AD as contributing etiologic

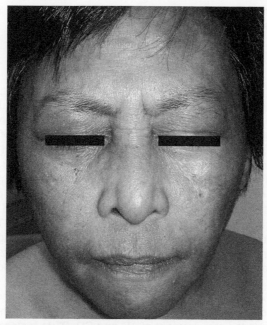

Fig. 1. Contact dermatitis of the eyelid and face in a patient with atopic dermatitis.

factor.[32] ICD commonly presents as a localized dermatitis without vesicles in webs of fingers; it extends onto the dorsal and ventral surfaces in an "apron" pattern, and includes the dorsum of the hands and palms, and the ball of the thumb. On the other hand, ACD often has vesicles, and favors the fingertips, nail folds, and dorsum of the hands, and, less commonly, involves the palms. ICD often precedes ACD; therefore, some pattern changes should prompt PT, such as increasing dermatitis from web spaces to fingertips or from palms to dorsal surfaces.[33]

Flexural Areas of Neck

Flexural areas of the neck are a common site of AD and CD. Common causes of CD in this area are irritant reactions to permanent waves ("perms"), hair dyes, shampoos, and conditioners, perfumes, nail polish, or nickel from necklaces or zippers.

Dermatitis with Scattered Generalized Distribution

Dermatitis with a generalized distribution is a difficult diagnostic challenge because it lacks the characteristic distribution that suggests a diagnosis of ACD. Generalized dermatitis also occurs in AD. The frequency of positive and relevant PT is unknown. Zug and colleagues[34] reported that approximately 15% of patients with positive PT results had scattered generalized dermatitis only, and approximately half (49%) had a positive PT reaction deemed at least possibly relevant to their dermatitis. The prevalence of scattered generalized dermatitis was higher in patients with a history of AD. However, 8% to 10% of patients with scattered generalized dermatitis remain in the unclassified eczema category. The two most common allergens identified were nickel and balsam of Peru. Other relevant positive PT reactions in this patient population include those to preservatives (formaldehyde, quaternium 15, methyldibromoglutaronitrile/phenoxyethanol, diazolidinyl urea, 2-bromo-2-nitropropane-1, 3-diol imidazolidinyl urea, and dimethyl-dimethyl hydantoin) and propylene glycol. Dyes such as Disperse Blue 106 in synthetic fibers in children's garments have also been implicated.[35]

SPECIFIC CONTACT ALLERGENS IN PATIENTS WITH AD
Topical Antibiotics/Antiseptics

Antibiotic topical preparations and antiseptics are often used as adjuncts in the treatment of AD. Jappe and colleagues[36] compared the frequency of sensitization to antibiotics and antiseptics in patients with both active AD and a history of AD versus those without active or previous history of AD. The allergens included were neomycin sulfate, gentamycin sulfate, erythromycin, fusidic acid, polymyxin B, oxytetracycline, nitrofurazone, framycetin, bacitracin, chloramphenicol, benzalkonium chloride, benzyl alcohol, triclosan, chlorhexidine, benzoate, formaldehyde, benzoyl peroxide, chloracetamide, and sulfacetamide. Results controlled for both age and sex did not find a higher risk among patients with AD than among those without. The investigators concluded that patients with AD had no increased risk of developing contact sensitization. A large number of patients with or without AD are sensitized to neomycin; atopy, old age, stasis dermatitis, and leg ulcers are significant risk factors for ACD to neomycin.

Triclosan is a biocide with antibacterial and antifungal activity through its disruption of cellular membranes used in dental, medical, cosmetic, and household products.[37] It has also been used in the management of AD and CD. PT to triclosan- and triclosan-containing creams was performed in addition to a standard series in 275 patients, of whom 55 had AD and 122 had ACD.[37] None of the 55 patients with AD had a positive PT reaction to triclosan, and only 6 (2.1%) of all patients tested positive for triclosan- or triclosan-containing products, reiterating a low incidence of contact sensitization especially in the atopic population. In a double-blind, prospective, randomized, controlled study, allergy to alcohol-based hand rubs was tested in patients with and without AD using an occlusive PT.[38] Tolerance to all five rubs was good among both populations, with no significant differences noted.

Topical Corticosteroids

Topical corticosteroid contact allergy affects 0.5% to 5.8% of patients.[39] Risk factors contributing to the development of delayed hypersensitivity to corticosteroids include chronic inflammatory skin disease (chronic venous leg ulcers [CVLUs], stasis dermatitis, CD), a history of two or more positive PT results, and multiple medicament sensitivities. In one study, 71 children with AD who used corticosteroids for at least 6 months underwent PT using a panel containing tixocortol pivalate 0.1%, budesonide 0.01%, hydrocortisone-17-butyrate 1%, and their own preparations, with readings made at days 2, 4, and 7.[40] Only one child had a positive reaction to tixocortol pivalate, hydrocortisone-17-butyrate, and Locoidon cream. These data are reassuring in that all corticosteroid groups were screened for, readings were conducted a week out, and personal products were also included.

ACD to topical corticosteroids was also assessed in a group of 140 adult patients with CVLUs (n = 50), AD (n = 30), and CD (n = 30).[39] These patients underwent PT using the European standard series, antibiotics, and corticosteroids. Overall positive PT results were seen in 80% of patients with CVLU and CD and 30% of those with AD; 40% of patients with CVLU were positive to corticosteroids versus 3% of those with AD and 20% of those with CD. The positive rate noted among the patients with AD is similar to rates attributed to corticosteroid allergy overall.

PT for corticosteroid allergy should include the groups of simultaneously or cross-reacting corticosteroids,[41] and the vehicle and preservatives in the preparations. Corticosteroids within a group show a sevenfold increase in frequency of positive PT reactions (**Box 1**). Cross-reactivity between groups A and D2 and groups B and D2 also has been reported.[42] However, 90% of contact allergy to steroids will be detected by screening with tixocortol pivalate, budesonide, and the patient's commercial steroid.[43,44] A late reading on day 7 is recommended when testing for corticosteroid allergy.[45]

Compositae

Sesquiterpene lactone is an important allergen in the compositae (asteraceae) family of plants that is responsible for ACD.[46] These plants are valued as medicinal and are used in herbal medicaments and cosmetics.[46] Compositae sensitization was traditionally believed to be highly prevalent in adults as an occupational disease in florists, farmers, and gardeners,[47] and in cosmetic dermatitis. However, case reports in the literature have included children with AD.[48] In one study in which 641 consecutive children and adolescents underwent PT with standard series and compositae mixed in 5% petrolatum, 17 children had positive reactions to this allergen.[47] Of these patients, 12 had AD, and the compositae allergy was either of current or past relevance. Because of higher prevalence of positive PT reactions to compositae in children with AD compared to those without ($P = .03$), the authors recommended using compositae mix when screening patients with AD experiencing airborne dermatitis.[47] In summary, contact sensitization to compositae should be suspected in patients with a personal or family history of atopy, and dermatitis exacerbated in summer with plant exposure.[48]

Dyes

New trends in permanent and temporary tattoos have emerged. Henna is used in multiple products, including hair dyes, shampoos, cosmetics, and temporary tattoos. It is obtained from the Lawsonia alba or inermis shrub cultivated in North Africa, India, and Sri Lanka,[49] with lawsone (a napthoquinone) considered the major allergen. With the addition of dyeing agents such as indigo, p-phenylenediamine (PPD), and/or diaminotoluenes, henna can impart hair colors other than the orange red from its unadulterated version.[49] An 11-year-old boy with an underlying history of AD and allergic rhinitis developed itch and edema 7 days after applying a temporary black henna tattoo on his right arm. A 4+ reaction to PPD was noted when the patient underwent PT using the European standard series. Although the exact compounds in the preparation used for the tattoo were unknown, the authors postulated that PPD was the allergen of importance because it is often present in henna at high concentrations.[49] PT using a panel of nine common allergens in a group of hairdressers with and without AD resulted in positive PT reactions in 60% of those with eczematous AD, 53% with asthma or allergic rhinitis, and 58% without AD.[50]

Nail Polish

Tosylamide/formaldehyde resin is a product added to nail polish to ensure good adhesion of polish to the nail bed.[51] It has been found to be clinically relevant in positive PT reactions in patients with eyelid dermatitis.[24] A 4-year-old girl with a history of AD was evaluated for new-onset eyelid dermatitis and worsening of flexural AD.[51] Her patch test showed a 1+ reaction to tosylamide/formaldehyde 10% in petroleum. Her history was consistent with the regular application of nail polish by a sibling. Once these products were discontinued the girl showed a significant improvement in symptoms.

Box 1
Structural groups of corticosteroids[a]

Class A (hydrocortisone and tixocortol pivalate: have C17 or C21 short-chain ester)

Hydrocortisone

Hydrocortisone acetate

Tixocortol

Prednisone

Prednisolone

Prednisolone acetate

Cloprednol

Cortisone

Cortisone acetate

Fludrocortisone

Methylprednisolone acetate

Class B (acetonides: have C16 C17 cis–ketal or –diol additions)

Triamcinolone acetonide

Budesonide

Desonide

Fluocinonide

Fluocinolone acetonide

Amcinonide

Halcinonide

Class C (nonesterified betamethasone: have C16 methyl group)

Betamethasone sodium phosphate

Dexamethasone

Dexamethasone sodium phosphate

Fluocortolone

Class D1 (C16 methyl group and halogenated B ring)

Clobetasone 17-butyrate

Clobetasone-17-propionate

Betamethasone-valerate

Betamethasone-dipropionate

Aclometasone dipropionate

Fluocortolone caproate

Fluocortolone-pivalate

Mometasone furoate

Class D2 (labile esters without C16 methyl or B ring halogen substitution)

Hydrocortisone 17-butyrate

Hydrocortisone-17-valerate

Hydrocortisone-17-aceponate

Hydrocortisone-17-buteprate

Methylprednisolone aceponate

[a] Cross-reactivity is based on two immune recognition sites: C 6/9 and C16/17 substitutions.

Latex

ACD to latex allergens is traditionally believed to be secondary to rubber chemicals (thiuram mix, mercapto mix) used in the manufacturing process.[52] Children suspected of having rubber ACD underwent PT using standardized rubber chemicals (thiuram, carba, and mercapto mix) in addition to a limited pediatric panel and natural rubber latex (NRL) allergen.[52] Of these children, 32 had positive reactions to both NRL preparation and personal rubber items but negative reactions to rubber chemicals. Of clinical significance, 30 of 32 patients had AD, with 2/3rds classified as mild to moderate AD and 1/3rd classified as severe AD according to SCORAD.[52] These patients with AD were also found to have other sensitizing contact allergens, positive prick tests to foods non–cross-reactive with NRL proteins, and inhalant allergen sensitization. Of these 32 children, 27 who had positive results to NRL who were retested 1 year later were still positive to this antigen.[52]

Makela and colleagues[53] evaluated ACD in patients with AD based on location of the dermatitis, dividing 801 patients with AD into 5 groups: hand dermatitis, facial dermatitis, hand and face dermatitis (HFD), dermatitis other than hands or face (OD), and patients without dermatitis (ND) but history of allergic rhinitis, allergic conjunctivitis, or asthma.[53] These patients underwent PT to 24 common contact allergens in the International Contact Dermatitis Research Group standard series. Nickel was the most common allergen in all groups, and fragrance mix and Balsam of Peru were especially common in the hand dermatitis group. After 16 years, these patients were sent a questionnaire inquiring about location and symptoms of dermatitis over the previous 2 weeks.[53] Responses showed that the number of patients in the hand dermatitis and OD groups decreased, those in the ND and HFD groups increased, and no change occurred in face dermatitis group.

PT for patients with AD is recommended for accurate identification of allergens that may be exacerbating the disease, particularly for topicals being used by the patient if they experience disease persistence or flaring despite appropriate therapy.[54] With positive PT results that are relevant, avoidance can be implemented and exacerbations may be curtailed.[54]

SUMMARY

CD is at least as common in patients with AD as in the general population, if not more. Thus, patients with AD should be considered for PT. Although conflicting data exist, the severity of the AD may impact the results obtained through PT. Younger patients with AD may yield more positive results on PT. Hand eczema and compositae allergy are more common in patients with AD. Reassuringly, PT is positive for antiseptic topicals and corticosteroids in only a small subset of patients. When personal products are patch tested, emollients should be included in the series.

REFERENCES

1. Bickers DR, Lim HW, Margolis D, et al. The burden of skin diseases: 2004 a joint project of the American Academy of Dermatology and the Society for Investigative Dermatology. J Am Acad Dermatol 2006;55:490–500.
2. Wolf R, Orion E, Matz H, et al. Still elusive relationship between atopic dermatitis and allergic contact dermatitis. Acta Dermatovenerol Croat 2003;11(4):247–50.
3. Leung DY, Boguniewicz M, Howell MD, et al. New insights into atopic dermatitis. J Clin Invest 2004;113(5):651–7.

4. Boguniewicz M, Leung DY. 10. Atopic dermatitis. J Allergy Clin Immunol 2006; 117(Suppl 2 Mini-Primer):S475–80.
5. Forsbeck M, Hovmark A, Skog E. Patch testing, tuberculin testing and sensitization with dinitrochlorobenzene and nitrosodimethylanilini of patients with atopic dermatitis. Acta Derm Venereol 1976;56(2):135–8.
6. Jones HE, Lewis CW, McMarlin SL. Allergic contact sensitivity in atopic dermatitis. Arch Dermatol 1973;107(2):217–22.
7. Palacios J, Fuller EW, Blaylock WK. Immunological capabilities of patients with atopic dermatitis. J Invest Dermatol 1966;47(5):484–90.
8. Candi E, Schmidt R, Melino G. The cornified envelope: a model of cell death in the skin. Nat Rev Mol Cell Biol 2005;6(4):328–40.
9. Novak N, Baurecht H, Schafer T, et al. Loss-of-function mutations in the filaggrin gene and allergic contact sensitization to nickel. J Invest Dermatol 2008;128(6): 1430–5.
10. Sonkoly E, Muller A, Lauerma AI, et al. IL-31: a new link between T cells and pruritus in atopic skin inflammation. J Allergy Clin Immunol 2006;117(2): 411–7.
11. Zhang Q, Putheti P, Zhou Q, et al. Structures and biological functions of IL-31 and IL-31 receptors. Cytokine Growth Factor Rev 2008;19(5–6):347–56.
12. Neis MM, Peters B, Dreuw A, et al. Enhanced expression levels of IL-31 correlate with IL-4 and IL-13 in atopic and allergic contact dermatitis. J Allergy Clin Immunol 2006;118(4):930–7.
13. Bilsborough J, Leung DY, Maurer M, et al. IL-31 is associated with cutaneous lymphocyte antigen-positive skin homing T cells in patients with atopic dermatitis. J Allergy Clin Immunol 2006;117(2):418–25.
14. Fartasch M, Schnetz E, Diepgen TL. Characterization of detergent-induced barrier alterations – effect of barrier cream on irritation. J Investig Dermatol Symp Proc 1998;3(2):121–7.
15. Wood LC, Jackson SM, Elias PM, et al. Cutaneous barrier perturbation stimulates cytokine production in the epidermis of mice. J Clin Invest 1992;90(2):482–7.
16. Krasteva M, Kehren J, Horand F, et al. Dual role of dendritic cells in the induction and down-regulation of antigen-specific cutaneous inflammation. J Immunol 1998;160(3):1181–90.
17. Giordano-Labadie F, Rance F, Pellegrin F, et al. Frequency of contact allergy in children with atopic dermatitis: results of a prospective study of 137 cases. Contact Dermatitis 1999;40(4):192–5.
18. Czarnobilska E, Obtulowicz K, Dyga W, et al. Contact hypersensitivity and allergic contact dermatitis among school children and teenagers with eczema. Contact Dermatitis 2009;60(5):264–9.
19. Sharma AD. Allergic contact dermatitis in patients with atopic dermatitis: a clinical study. Indian J Dermatol Venereol Leprol 2005;71(2):96–8.
20. Hanifin JM, Rajka G. Diagnostic features of atopic dermatitis. Acta Derm Venereol 1980;92S:44–7.
21. Belhadjali H, Mohamed M, Youssef M, et al. Contact sensitization in atopic dermatitis: results of a prospective study of 89 cases in Tunisia. Contact Dermatitis 2008;58(3):188–9.
22. Uehara M, Sawai T. A longitudinal study of contact sensitivity in patients with atopic dermatitis. Arch Dermatol 1989;125(3):366–8.
23. Mailhol C, Lauwers-Cances V, Rance F, et al. Prevalence and risk factors for allergic contact dermatitis to topical treatment in atopic dermatitis: a study in 641 children. Allergy 2009;64(5):801–6.

24. Beattie PE, Green C, Lowe G, et al. Which children should we patch test? Clin Exp Dermatol 2007;32(1):6–11.
25. Mortz CG, Lauritsen JM, Bindslev-Jensen C, et al. Prevalence of atopic dermatitis, asthma, allergic rhinitis, and hand and contact dermatitis in adolescents. The Odense Adolescence Cohort Study on Atopic Diseases and Dermatitis. Br J Dermatol 2001;144(3):523–32.
26. Ingordo V, D'Andria G, D'Andria C, et al. Clinical relevance of contact sensitization in atopic dermatitis. Contact Dermatitis 2001;45(4):239–40.
27. Ayala F, Fabbrocini G, Bacchilega R, et al. Eyelid dermatitis: an evaluation of 447 patients. Am J Contact Dermat 2003;14(2):69–74.
28. Rietschel RL, Warshaw EM, Sasseville D, et al. Common contact allergens associated with eyelid dermatitis: data from the North American Contact Dermatitis Group 2003-2004 study period. Dermatitis 2007;18(2):78–81.
29. Guin JD. Eyelid dermatitis: experience in 203 cases. J Am Acad Dermatol 2002; 47(5):755–65.
30. Valsecchi R, Imberti G, Martino D, et al. Eyelid dermatitis: an evaluation of 150 patients. Contact Dermatitis 1992;27(3):143–7.
31. Zug KA, Kornik R, Belsito DV, et al. Patch-testing North American lip dermatitis patients: data from the North American Contact Dermatitis Group, 2001 to 2004. Dermatitis 2008;19(4):202–8.
32. Simpson EL, Thompson MM, Hanifin JM. Prevalence and morphology of hand eczema in patients with atopic dermatitis. Dermatitis 2006;17(3):123–7.
33. Warshaw E, Lee G, Storrs FJ. Hand dermatitis: a review of clinical features, therapeutic options, and long-term outcomes. Am J Contact Dermat 2003;14(3):119–37.
34. Zug KA, Rietschel RL, Warshaw EM, et al. The value of patch testing patients with a scattered generalized distribution of dermatitis: retrospective cross-sectional analyses of North American Contact Dermatitis Group data, 2001 to 2004. J Am Acad Dermatol 2008;59(3):426–31.
35. Seidenari S, Giusti F, Pepe P, et al. Contact sensitization in 1094 children undergoing patch testing over a 7-year period. Pediatr Dermatol 2005;22(1):1–5.
36. Jappe U, Schnuch A, Uter W. Frequency of sensitization to antimicrobials in patients with atopic eczema compared with nonatopic individuals: analysis of multicentre surveillance data, 1995–1999. Br J Dermatol 2003;149(1):87–93.
37. Schena D, Papagrigoraki A, Girolomoni G. Sensitizing potential of triclosan and triclosan-based skin care products in patients with chronic eczema. Dermatol Ther 2008;21(Suppl 2):S35–8.
38. Kampf G, Wigger-Alberti W, Wilhelm KP. Do atopics tolerate alcohol-based hand rubs? A prospective, controlled, randomized double-blind clinical trial. Acta Derm Venereol 2006;86(2):140–3.
39. Zmudzinska M, Czarnecka-Operacz M, Silny W. Contact allergy to glucocorticosteroids in patients with chronic venous leg ulcers, atopic dermatitis and contact allergy. Acta Dermatovenerol Croat 2008;16(2):72–8.
40. Foti C, Bonifazi E, Casulli C, et al. Contact allergy to topical corticosteroids in children with atopic dermatitis. Contact Dermatitis 2005;52(3):162–3.
41. Lepoittevin JP, Drieghe J, Dooms-Goossens A. Studies in patients with corticosteroid contact allergy. Understanding cross-reactivity among different steroids. Arch Dermatol 1995;131(1):31–7.
42. Wilkinson SM. Corticosteroid cross-reactions: an alternative view. Contact Dermatitis 2000;42(2):59–63.
43. Bjarnason B, Flosadottir E, Fischer T. Assessment of budesonide patch tests. Contact Dermatitis 1999;41(4):211–7.

44. Boffa MJ, Wilkinson SM, Beck MH. Screening for corticosteroid contact hypersensitivity. Contact Dermatitis 1995;33(3):149–51.
45. McFadden J. Contact allergic reactions in patients with atopic eczema. Acta Derm Venereol Suppl (Stockh) 2005;(215):28–32.
46. Paulsen E. Contact sensitization from Compositae-containing herbal remedies and cosmetics. Contact Dermatitis 2002;47(4):189–98.
47. Belloni Fortina A, Romano I, Peserico A. Contact sensitization to Compositae mix in children. J Am Acad Dermatol 2005;53(5):877–80.
48. Paulsen E, Otkjaer A, Andersen KE. Sesquiterpene lactone dermatitis in the young: is atopy a risk factor? Contact Dermatitis 2008;59(1):1–6.
49. Corrente S, Moschese V, Chianca M, et al. Temporary henna tattoo is unsafe in atopic children. Acta Paediatr 2007;96(3):469–71.
50. Sutthipisal N, McFadden JP, Cronin E. Sensitization in atopic and non-atopic hairdressers with hand eczema. Contact Dermatitis 1993;29(4):206–9.
51. Jacob SE, Stechschulte SA. Tosylamide/formaldehyde resin allergy–a consideration in the atopic toddler. Contact Dermatitis 2008;58(5):312–3.
52. Guillet G, Guillet MH, Dagregorio G. Allergic contact dermatitis from natural rubber latex in atopic dermatitis and the risk of later Type I allergy. Contact Dermatitis 2005;53(1):46–51.
53. Makela L, Lammintausta K, Kalimo K. Contact sensitivity and atopic dermatitis: association with prognosis, a follow-up study in 801 atopic patients. Contact Dermatitis 2007;56(2):76–80.
54. Vender RB. The utility of patch testing children with atopic dermatitis. Skin Therapy Lett 2002;7(6):4–6.

Evolution of Conventional Therapy in Atopic Dermatitis

Andreas Wollenberg, MD[a],*, Christina Schnopp, MD[b]

KEYWORDS

- Atopic dermatitis • Therapy • Glucocorticosteroids
- Calcineurin inhibitors • Emollients

Therapy of atopic dermatitis (AD) is an ever-changing field. Innovations and pseudoinnovations regarding topical therapy, trends in public knowledge, and awareness of drug risks and benefits as well as evolving understanding of the immunobiologic mechanisms underlying AD contribute to the ongoing evolution in therapy. Because most currently used treatment options for patients with AD may be classified as targeting primarily either skin barrier, microbial colonization, infection or inflammation of AD, the authors have chosen to follow this classification in this review.

One hundred years ago, topical therapy of AD consisted largely of the black and malodorous coal tar preparations that only senior colleagues are likely to recall from clinical practice. The low acceptance of the various tar preparations by most patients, together with experimental evidence of an increased carcinogenic risk, reduced the clinical use of tar products to a minimum. One relevant exception is sulfonated shale oil preparations, because these are well tolerated and not considered carcinogenic.[1] The antiproliferative and anti-inflammatory effects of these drugs are synergistic with topical corticosteroids (TCSs) in the treatment of prurigo nodularis.

Anti-inflammatory treatment options for AD have been revolutionized during the twentieth century by the introduction of two new drug classes into clinical practice—TCSs and topical calcineurin inhibitors (TCIs). The topical anti-inflammatory drugs used today include a wide variety of TCS formulations and two different TCI drugs.[2]

THERAPY-RELEVANT PATHOGENIC ASPECTS OF ATOPIC DERMATITIS

The disease-defining clinical phenotype of AD includes highly pruritic, eczematous skin lesions preferentially affecting the large body folds, head and neck region,

[a] Department of Dermatology and Allergy, Ludwig-Maximilian University, Frauenlobstrasse 9-11, D-80331 Munich, Germany
[b] Department of Dermatology and Allergy, Technical University, Biedersteinerstrasse 29, D-80802 Munich, Germany
* Corresponding author.
E-mail address: wollenberg@lrz.uni-muenchen.de

Immunol Allergy Clin N Am 30 (2010) 351–368
doi:10.1016/j.iac.2010.06.005
0889-8561/10/$ – see front matter © 2010 Published by Elsevier Inc.

immunology.theclinics.com

dryness of uninvolved skin, and a lymphohistiocytic infiltrate with some extent of spongiosis. Some experts delineate a clinically more severe extrinsic subtype associated with IgE responses to allergens and a tendency towards cutaneous infections from a clinically milder, intrinsic phenotype lacking these features.[3] The genetic background of AD involves variants of immune function genes as well as barrier function genes.[4] Both are discussed briefly, as far as they are of therapeutic relevance.

EPIDERMAL BARRIER DYSFUNCTION IN ATOPIC DERMATITIS

Dryness of clinically uninvolved skin is a diagnostic feature of AD as well as a severity marker of the disease.[5] The identification of filaggrin (FLG) mutations as the genetic basis of ichthyosis vulgaris, which is a risk factor for AD, has renewed interest in epidermal barrier dysfunction of patients with AD.[6,7] Epidermal barrier function is localized primarily in the stratum corneum and consists mainly of corneocytes with a cornified envelope and lipid-enriched intercellular domains.[7]

FLG is produced in stratum granulosum of the epidermis and plays an important role in the terminal differentiation of keratinocytes to anucleate corneocytes. Furthermore, FLG degradation products include amino acids, which contribute to the composition of natural moisturizing factor in the stratum corneum.[8,9] Whereas homozygous mutations in the FLG gene cause severe manifestations of ichthyosis vulgaris,[10] 25% to 30% of patients with AD are heterozygous for FLG compared with 7% to 8% in the overall population.[11–13] A decreased stratum corneum hydration, presumably caused by a lack of natural moisturizing factor, and an increased skin pH in FLG mutation carriers seem crucial for the barrier defect of AD.[7] The idea that impaired barrier function leads to increased outside-inside permeability and enhanced penetration of allergens is intruiging.[14,15]

So-called barrier lipids are produced by keratinocytes from stratum basale to stratum granulosum, stored intracellularly in lamellar bodies, and are finally excreted to the extracellular space. Epidermal lipids are mainly composed of ceramides (approximately 50%), cholesterol (approximately 25%), free fatty acids (10%–15%), and cholesterol sulfate (<5%)—independent of nutritional factors.[16] Patients with AD produce fewer and different lipids in their epidermal layers.[17] Ceramide composition seems to be specifically altered compared with healthy controls and other skin diseases.[18] An abnormal function of a sphingomyelin deacylase may lead to higher ceramide degradation.[19,20]

In summary, addressing epidermal barrier dysfunction is a logical way of treating AD, and current knowledge about epidermal barrier dysfunction in AD suggests basic therapy with a lipid-rich emollient, ideally containing ceramides and moisturizers, thus compensating for known AD-specific deficiencies.

COLONIZATION AND INFECTION IN ATOPIC DERMATITIS

The characteristic atopic immune dysregulation involves a tendency to colonization and infection with staphylococci as well as a reduced innate immune response, especially against viral infections[21] (see the article by Ong and Leung elsewhere in this issue for further exploration of this topic). Eczema herpeticum, which is the disseminated infection of eczema lesions with herpes simplex virus, occurs almost exclusively in patients with AD.[22] In addition, AD lesions are heavily colonized with *Staphylococcus aureus* known to produce exotoxins (**Fig. 1**), which may act as antigens or superantigens.[23] Thus, not only staphylococcal infections but also colonization of AD with *S aureus* needs to be therapeutically addressed.

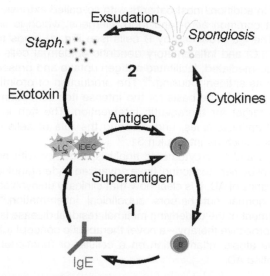

Fig. 1. IgE-mediated antigen presentation and immunoactivation by staphylococcal super-antigens. An antigen-specific vicious circle of IgE-mediated antigen presentation by Langerhans cells (LC) or inflammatory dendritic epidermal cells (IDEC) to T cells (1) interacts with an unspecific, superantigen-driven vicious circle activating all T cells sharing the same T-cell receptor family (2).

Production of antimicrobial peptides, some of which are upregulated on cutaneous inflammation, is a powerful mechanism of the innate immune system for fighting invading microorganisms, such as bacteria, fungi, and viruses, after damage of the epithelial surface.[24] A single cathelicidin and several defensins have been characterized in humans. The demonstration of deficient upregulation of the antimicrobial peptides, human β-defensin (HBD)-2 and human cathelicidin LL-37, in skin lesions of AD stimulated research in this field.[25] Whereas HBD-1 is constitutively expressed by keratinocytes, proinflammatory stimuli induce the expression of HBD-2, HBD-3, and the cathelicidin LL-37.[26]

Preferential adherence by different surface-associated proteins[27,28] and impaired defense factors in atopic individuals, including reduced defensin expression and polymorphisms in pattern recognition receptors,[29,30] favor S aureus colonization of atopic skin. Clinical and experimental data suggest that S aureus is a distinct aggravation factor for AD. Among other virulence factors, many of the S aureus strains isolated from AD produce superantigens, which continuously stimulate the host immune system and thereby contribute to chronification and exacerbation of skin symptoms.[4] In addition, S aureus colonization induces production of specific IgE antibodies to staphylococcal components, especially superantigens, which may further aggravate clinical symptoms.[31,32]

In summary, colonization and infection of the skin must be considered if treating patients with AD on a long-term basis. A reduction of the staphylococcal burden may be as important for patients as treating clinically infected AD skin.

CUTANEOUS INFLAMMATION IN ATOPIC DERMATITIS

The clinical definition of AD is based on the presence of cutaneous inflammation, and the inflammatory infiltrate of AD consists of activated lymphocytes and histiocytic cells.[33] In addition, most patients with so-called extrinsic AD develop IgE responses against common aero- and food allergens, which is also a diagnostic feature of AD.[34] The IgE produced by B cells (see **Fig. 1**) binds to the surface of Langerhans cells (LC) and inflammatory dendritic epidermal cells (IDEC),[35] where it contributes to IgE-mediated, facilitated antigen uptake and presentation, a mechanism also known as antigen focusing.[36] The production of proinflammatory cytokines by lesional T cells is the basis for the intense itch sensation in patients with AD and is a key target for therapeutic intervention. The itch in AD in not well controlled by oral antihistamines, underscoring the role of cells other than mast cells and mediators, such as interleukin 31.[37]

Immunohistologic and flow cytometric analysis, together with noninvasive techniques for epidermal barrier monitoring, have advanced understanding of the immunobiologic characteristics of AD. It is clear now that clinically uninvolved skin of patients with AD is not normal but harbors subclinical inflammation.[38] Minimal anti-inflammatory treatment of the underlying minimal, residual disease is the immunobiologic rationale for proactive therapy—a novel therapeutic concept (discussed later).[39] Interfering with the atopic inflammation on a cellular or functional level is another logical way of treating AD.

EMOLLIENT USE AND BASIC THERAPY OF ATOPIC DERMATITIS

Emollients are used to restore disrupted epidermal barrier function in AD. The choice of an oil-in-water or water-in-oil emulsion depends on the actual skin condition. Emollients with low fat content are favorable for highly inflamed, oozing lesions, whereas chronic, dry eczematous lesions should be treated with fat-containing emollients. Ointments with high fat content or hydrophilic gels containing almost no fat should be avoided.[40] The choice of the emollient should be adapted with flares and seasonal climatic conditions (**Box 1**). Gycerol and urea are the most commonly used moisturizers. In vivo studies in healthy volunteers have shown that 10% glycerol is more effective than 5% glycerol, whereas 10% urea did not show advantages compared with 5% urea.[41,42]

Box 1
Algorithm for choice of topical therapy

1. Describe the skin changes

↓

2. Determine the diagnosis (or rank differential diagnoses)

↓

3. Define aims of therapy

↓

4. Choose active ingredients and vehicle system

↓

5. Decide on commercial product or compounding

An expert dermatologist's algorithm for choice of topical therapy is complex and typically follows the steps of description, diagnosis, choice of active ingredients, and vehicle system to reach the therapeutic goal and choice between commercial products or traditional compounding.

Although most experts in and guidelines for AD treatment emphasize the importance of regular emollient use in AD,[43,44] there are only a few studies proving this effect. A recent study compared morning use of an emollient and evening use of an oil bath with no basic therapy at all over 6 weeks.[45] Additionally, a mild topical corticosteroid was applied on eczematous lesions during the first 2 weeks. The basic therapy group showed only slight worsening of their skin condition (measured by EASI, the "eczema area and severity index"), whereas the control group showed significant deterioration of their AD at days 28 and 42, almost reaching the start values of EASI. Other studies have shown that regular basic therapy reduces signs and symptoms of AD with less or equal consumption of TCIs.[46,47] A new formulation recently developed for correction of lipid biochemical abnormalities in AD has been shown to be noninferior to fluticasone propionate cream with respect to pruritus and sleep loss as well as reduction in SCORAD, the "scoring atopic dermatitis" score over a 28-day period in a randomized multicenter study in 121 patients with AD.[48] Experimental data further suggest that regular use of topical glucocorticosteroids can lead to disruption of epidermal barrier function by inhibiting epidermal synthesis of fatty acids.[49] This effect can be alleviated by application of a mixture of ceramides, free fatty acids, and cholesterol,[50] further supporting regular use of appropriate emollients.

Effectiveness of basic therapy is directly linked to patient adherence to a regular application schedule and, therefore, cosmetic acceptance of an emollient is crucial. Doctors should ask their patients if they are happy with qualities, such as texture, dispersion, permeation, and scent, of their emollient and assist in choosing acceptable products.

ANTIMICROBIAL TREATMENT IN ATOPIC DERMATITIS

Lesional and nonlesional AD skin is uniquely colonized with S aureus, which is the most important target for antimicrobial therapy in patients with AD. Several studies have determined colonization rates with S aureus as high as 90% of all analyzed patients.[23,51,52] Even with extensive antimicrobial treatment, eradication of S aureus is only transient, with recurrence rates of almost 100%.[53–55]

S aureus infection is the most common complication of AD and is associated with more severe skin lesions.[56] Impetiginized AD is diagnosed clinically, based on oozing and formation of yellowish crusts. Detection of S aureus is not diagnostic for impetiginization of AD because of high colonization rates and exact quantitative analyses are not routinely performed. Bacterial culture prior to therapy is important, however, to be able to adjust primary antibiotic treatment if necessary and detect methicillin-resistant S aureus, Streptococcus pyogenes, or other bacteria that might be additionally involved.

Although systemic antibiotics are used in treatment interventions, antiseptics are used in the long-term management of patients with AD to prevent infection or reduce bacterial counts. Amelioration of inflammation through anti-inflammatory treatment with topical steroids or TCIs also results in reduced bacterial numbers.[57,58]

Some studies have shown that intensive antibacterial treatment of AD leads to a significant amelioration of AD,[53] whereas others did not.[55,59] In general, there was no sustained effect.

A recent Cochrane Database report analyzing the "small and poorly reported" studies on antistaphylococcal intervention in patients with AD concluded that there was insufficient evidence for adding antibacterial treatment to anti-inflammatory regimens in AD,[60] but this approach may be clinically useful in selected patients.

TOPICAL TREATMENT OF AD WITH ANTIBIOTICS

Topical formulations of antibiotics for treatment of S aureus–colonized AD lesions have been tested in clinical trials alone or in combination with glucocorticosteroids, but the results for mupirocin 2%, fusidic acid 2%, and tetracycline 3% were conflicting.[61–63] Because topical use of antibiotics may induce bacterial resistance and contact allergy, topical antibiotics should not be used as first-line treatments in AD. The anatomic and physiological peculiarities of the eyelid region allow one exception of this rule, which is the ophthalmic use of fusidic acid gel 1% in addition to topical anti-inflammatory treatment.[2] Whether or not new classes of antibiotics, such as the pleuromutilins,[64] will enter clinical routine use must be awaited.

TOPICAL TREATMENT OF AD WITH ANTISEPTICS

The main advantages of antiseptics over antibiotics are their much lower potential to induce resistance in S aureus strains with repeated use, the availability of different preparations, and their low risk for inducing contact allergy. Topical antiseptics are indicated in conjunction with systemic antibiotic treatment for severely impetiginized AD as well as for long-term adjunct therapy in patients with recurring clinical superinfection due to S aureus. Furthermore, antiseptics have been proposed as part of long-term antibacterial therapy in patients with S aureus colonization to reduce potential proinflammatory stimuli.

Antiseptics are used in addition to systemic antibiotics to rapidly and effectively remove crusts and bacterial load from impetiginized AD lesions and include potassium permanganate ($KMnO_4$), sodium hypochlorie, triclosan, and chlorhexidine gluconate. It is important to carefully check for correct concentrations, because most antiseptics are toxic or at least irritating in higher concentrations.

Prophylactic antiseptic treatment is often recommended for patients with frequent bacterial infection, although there are no data from controlled trials to prove the effect. An antiseptic ointment can be compounded containing 1% to 2% triclosan or 0.5% to 1% chlorhexidine gluconate to be used for the whole body or the critical regions only. Prophylactic antiseptic baths twice weekly are another option for follow-up treatment of patients with AD after initial S aureus eradication.

Triclosan (2,4,4'-trichloro-2'-hydroxydiphenyl ether) is a lyophilic chlorophenol biocide with a broad-spectrum antibacterial activity, highly active against S aureus, Klebsiella pneumonia, and Proteus, with less to no effect on Pseudomonas, β-hemolytic streptococci, and Enterococci.[65] In dermatology, 1% to 3% triclosan is used as antibacterial therapy, and resistance has rarely been observed.[66] The lipophilic compound triclosan is suitable for water-in-oil formulations and frequently added to emollients.

Considerable amounts (6.3% in an in vitro system) of triclosan penetrate the skin but are readily excreted, predominantly by feces.[67] Triclosan has been found in breast milk from lactating mothers using ordinary cosmetic products,[68] but the levels were far lower than the no-observed-adverse-effect level (NOAEL).[69]

A randomized study from Singapore evaluated efficacy and safety of 1% triclosan ointment over a 27-day treatment period in mild to moderate AD (n = 60). Patients were allowed to use betamethasone valerate 0.025% cream as additional treatment. The triclosan group improved better in SCORAD, but the effect was significant on day 14 only and not on day 27. Topical glucocorticoid use, however, was reduced to half in the triclosan group ($P<.05$) indicating a steroid-sparing potential of the triclosan-containing emollient.[70] Other formulations have also been shown to be clinically effective (reviewed by Birnie and colleagues[60]).

Chlorhexidine gluconate, a biguanide, is widely used as an antiseptic in hand washes, oral hygiene products, and disinfectant for medical procedures. Its bactericidal activity to S aureus, low irritation potential, and suitability for use as bath wash or additive in oil-in-water formulations 0.5% to 1% led to topical use in patients with AD.

The only study published in patients with AD showed chlorhexidine baths equal to potassium permanganate baths in reducing severity of AD and S aureus colonization.[71] The in vitro activity of chlorhexidine gluconate (1/1000) against S aureus is significantly higher than $KMnO_4$ (1/10).[71] Several cases of severe immediate-type allergic reactions to chlorhexidine have been reported, and specific IgE antibodies were detectable in most patients affected.[72–74]

$KMnO_4$, a strong oxidizing compound, has been used for many years and gives a concentration-dependent, purple-pinkish color if dissolved in water. As a rule, $KMnO_4$ should always be thoroughly diluted to get a light pink color, because higher concentrations can cause necrosis of the skin. Because equally effective and safer alternatives exist, the authors do not recommend home treatment with $KMnO_4$.

Twice-weekly, full-body baths in diluted sodium hypochlorite (diluted bleach) have been shown effective for maintenance treatment after S aureus eradication in patients with AD.[75] After 14 days of open-label oral cephalexin treatment, 31 pediatric patients were randomly assigned to intermittent topical mupirocin intranasally (5 days per month) and sodium hypochlorite baths (final concentration 0.005%) twice weekly or petrolatum ointment and plain water baths for 3 months. EASI scores were reduced in the treatment group after 1 month ($P = .17$) and 3 months ($P = .004$) compared with placebo. Only the body parts submerged during bathing improved but not the head and neck area. As S aureus colonization was not quantified, it remains unclear whether or not the clinical effect of bleach baths can be explained by S aureus reduction on lesional skin or the astringent effects of the bleach baths.

Octenidine dihydrochloride 0.1% is mostly used in combination with phenoxyethanol 2% for disinfection of skin and mucous membranes. It is licensed for intermittent use in all age groups. In patients with AD, octenidine solution may be useful for wet antiseptic dressings in localized infected AD or antiseptic washes.

Povidone-iodine is a stable chemical complex of polyvinylpyrrolidone (povidone) and elemental iodine. Investigators in Japan have advocated 10% povidone-iodine solution as an antiseptic wash or bath for patients with AD,[76–78] but the potential local and systemic (thyroid function) side-effects limit the use of this substance.

FUTURE PROSPECTS ON ANTIMICROBIAL TREATMENT

Because eradication of S aureus on atopic skin is not feasible for longer periods, reductive measures for S aureus colonization in AD must be judged against their long-term side effects. Current data on systemic absorption with extensive use of antiseptic substances in patients with severely compromised skin barrier is not sufficient to formally exclude potential side effects. Alternatively, the effectiveness of adjuvant antiseptic treatment is clinically evident. The degree of skin inflammation seems the most important factor for bacterial load on AD skin. The data published so far do not justify the general addition of antibacterial measures to anti-inflammatory therapy.

In conclusion, the authors recommend an addition of antiseptics to the emollient or baths on a regular basis independent of clinical infection only for patients with special manifestations of AD (eg, weepy-type AD), special circumstances (eg, mothers of small babies), or elevated risk for systemic infection (eg, in-dwelling catheters or chronic wounds). Textiles with antiseptic properties (silver-coated textiles or alkoxysilane quarternary ammonium [AEGIS]-coated silk) might present a useful alternative for these patients.[79–81]

ANTI-INFLAMMATORY THERAPY OF ATOPIC DERMATITIS

Anti-inflammatory therapy is a mainstay of conventional management of AD along with epidermal barrier repair and anti-infective therapies (discussed previously). At present, there are only two important therapeutic classes in clinical use: TCSs and TCIs. The authors believe that the choice of therapeutic class should primarily follow the anatomic and physiological specificities of the affected region to be treated.[2]

ANTI-INFLAMMATORY THERAPY WITH CORTICOSTEROIDS

TCSs are widely regarded as first line anti-inflammatory treatment for AD and have traditionally been applied on inflamed skin according to patient needs.[82] Many corticosteroids with different therapeutic strengths are available in a variety of formulations. Their anti-inflammatory effects in AD have been well known for many years, but well-controlled studies are available for selected modern products only. With mild disease activity, small amounts of TCS in combination with liberal use of emollients are sufficient to maintain an acceptable skin status and do not produce adverse systemic or local effects.[2]

TCSs are grouped by potency, the classification differing between the United States and Europe. The local classification should be known to prescribers, because potent and very potent TCSs are more likely to cause depression of adrenal function than the mild and moderate potency products.[83]

Potent TCSs reduce inflammation faster than milder TCS preparations, thus leading to less inflammation-derived barrier defects. Alternatively, TCSs are known to damage the epidermal barrier by interfering with epidermal proliferation and differentiation process, thus leading to concerns especially in long-term use of the more potent substances.[7]

Tapering of TCS is a clinical need and should only be started once the erythema and itch have stopped. A reduction of application frequency as well as changing to a less potent substance are well established strategies protecting against withdrawal rebound.[84] The most useful way to spare steroids and avoid steroid-related side effects is not to spare them during acute flares but to combine baseline emollient skin care with an early anti-inflammatory intervention.[2] Clinical reality teaches that this ideal form of treatment may not be followed by the majority of patients.[85]

ANTI-INFLAMMATORY THERAPY WITH TOPICAL CALCINEURIN INHIBITORS

There are two TCIs, tacrolimus ointment and pimecrolimus cream, licensed for topical AD treatment in the United States and Europe. Many aspects of these drugs have been reviewed during the past years,[86] and the efficacy of both formulations has been demonstrated against placebo in clinical trials.[87,88] The anti-inflammatory potency of 0.1% tacrolimus ointment is similar to a corticosteroid with intermediate potency,[89] whereas 1.0% pimecrolimus cream is less effective.[90]

Safety issues of both TCIs have been assessed in many clinical trials, demonstrating the safety of these drugs in daily routine use.[2,91] The most frequently observed side effect is a transient burning sensation at the application site during the first few days of application.[87] It usually starts approximately 5 minutes after the application of the drug and may last up to 1 hour, but intensity and duration decrease almost completely within 1 week. Patients stay in a burning-free state if the application frequency is reduced to twice-weekly treatment.[92] Single cases of generalized viral infections, such as eczema herpeticum or eczema molluscatum, have been observed during TCI treatment,[93,94] but many controlled clinical trials have failed to demonstrate an increased frequency.

In contrast to TCSs, TCIs do not cause skin atrophy, thus favoring their use over TCSs in sensitive body areas.[95,96] Long-term anti-inflammatory treatment with TCIs is, therefore, preferred over TCSs on the face, eyelids, perioral region, genital area, axillary region, or inguinal folds.[2] Clinical and preclinical data do not indicate an increased risk for lymphoma induction over a period of 6 years or for photocarcinogenicity with TCI treatment.[97,98] Because the continuous administration of the systemic calcineurin inhibitor, cyclosporine, is associated with increased photocarcinogenicity risk in solid organ transplant patients, UV protection with proper clothing and topical sunscreen preparations is also advisable for patients with AD treated with TCIs. The use of TCIs under wet wraps or on erosive lesions may increase systemic absorption.

Tacrolimus ointment is potent enough to allow long-term monotherapy in children and adults.[92,99,100] Pimecrolimus cream has been studied for treatment of facial AD in children aged 2 to 11 years, showing good efficacy and safety.[101] Both TCIs are approved in the United States and Europe from 2 years of age and above.

PROACTIVE VERSUS REACTIVE THERAPY OF AD

Anti-inflammatory topical therapy has traditionally been administered to AD lesions only and was stopped or tapered down once visible lesions had cleared.[82] This traditional, reactive approach has in the past years been challenged by the proactive treatment concept, which is defined as a combination of predefined, long-term, anti-inflammatory treatment applied to previously affected areas of skin in combination with liberal use of emollients.[39] The proactive, usually twice-weekly, treatment regimen is started after all lesions have successfully been treated by an intensive, usually twice-daily treatment approach in addition to ongoing emollient therapy for previously unaffected skin.[102] Clinical trial data are available for few TCS products for up to 4 months as well as for tacrolimus ointment for a whole year.

The rationale for this approach is that that nonlesional, normal-looking skin of patients with AD is not normal but shows a barrier defect—the transepidermal water loss and the hydration of the stratum corneum of nonlesional AD skin are not normal but shown to be between normal human skin and lesional AD skin.[103] Increased permeability of nonlesional AD skin for protein allergens is important for the atopy patch test,[104] where protein allergens dissolved in petrolatum penetrate the epidermal barrier and elicit an eczematous skin reaction.[105] Extractable long-chain fatty acids essential for skin barrier function are reduced not only in lesional AD skin (75%) but also in nonlesional AD skin (60%).[106] This constitutive component of barrier defect adds to an inflammation-induced component.[107] The histology of nonlesional AD skin shows features of mild disease with a low-grade inflammatory infiltrate, swelling of endothelial cells, and thickening of the basement membrane zone.[33] Epidermal LC carrying IgE bound to the high-affinity IgE-receptor have been detected by immunohistochemistry in lesional and nonlesional AD skin but not in normal skin from nonatopic individuals.[108–111] Quantitative flow cytometry showed that LC express significantly more high-affinity IgE-receptors on the cell surface in nonlesional AD skin than in normal human skin.[112] In conclusion, there is overwhelming evidence that normal-looking, nonlesional AD skin is not normal at all but characterized by a clinically meaningful barrier function defect and a subclinical eczematous skin reaction.

Proactive therapy with topical tacrolimus ointment has been shown to reduce the number of flares, increase the number of flare-free days, and lead to an overall better skin status in children and adults.[92,100] Moreover, proactively treated patients reported a better quality of life during the entire 1-year trial compared with reactive therapy.[92] These results were unexpectedly achieved with a lower mean daily ointment use in the proactive treatment arm[113] and confirmed in a US trial with a 3-times weekly regimen.[114] The cost effectiveness of proactive therapy with topical tacrolimus has also been shown in a recent study.[113] There are no data for proactive therapy with pimecrolimus cream.

Proactive therapy with TCSs has also been investigated, and proactive fluticasone propionate treatment has been shown effective in a proactive approach in a few well controlled, short-term studies.[115,116] In addition, a single study using methylprednisolone aceponate has also shown the efficacy of the proactive approach for flare prevention.[117]

Proactive therapy may be regarded the superior treatment concept in moderate to severe AD, because objective and subjective efficacy parameters indicate fewer flares and better clinical efficacy of the anti-inflammatory medications applied to the patients. In daily practice, the pros and cons of both approaches should be explained and discussed with patients individually in order to reach an informed decision.[38]

SUBSTANCES WITH LOW OR UNPROVED ANTI-INFLAMMATORY POTENTIAL

There is a wide range of alternative, nonsteroidal, nonimmunosuppressive topical treatments with low or unproved anti-inflammatory potential (see the article by Lee and Bielory elsewhere in this issue for further exploration of this topic). These include tannins, zinc oxide, polidocanol, bufexamac, and phytotherapeutics, such as black cumin (*Nigella sativa*), witch hazel (*Hamamelis virginiana*), German camomile (*Matricaria chamomila*), St. John's wort (*Hypericum perforatum*), marigold (*Calendula officinalis*), bittersweet (*Solanum dulcamara*), and evening primrose oil (*Oenothera biennis*). Most of these substances have never been evaluated in clinical studies in patients with AD.

Tannins, zinc oxide, and polidocanol are widely used for their antipruritic effect, although controlled studies are lacking. They seem to be effective in a subgroup of patients and—because side effects are negligible—worth a trial. Tannins and zinc oxide have an additional astringed and possibly mild anti-inflammatory effect.

Bufexamac is no longer recommended in AD treatment because of its potential to elict severe contact dermatitis. Although sensitization rates in patients with AD in general do not differ from other patient groups, sensitization to bufexamac is 3 times higher in patients with AD.[118] In children, bufexamac is among the 10 most frequently diagnosed contact allergens, with a sensitization rate of 4.6%.[119]

St. John's wort, standardized to hyperforin 1.5% ointment, has shown a significant beneficial effect compared with placebo in a controlled study in patients with AD.[120] Because commercial preparations contain *Hypericum* in concentrations much lower than 1.5%, the effectivity of these products remains unclear. Hypericin, which is the phototoxic component in St. John's wort, has been eliminated in these preparations.

Evening primrose oil has been evaluated as topical treatment and nutritional supplement in several studies. A systematic review concluded that a beneficial effect of evening primrose oil in the treatment of AD has not been shown—even if theory predicts that these drugs could be effective.[121]

> **Box 2**
> **The Munich left hand rule for assessing new treatment**
>
> 1. Has the novel treatment been described exactly?
> 2. Is there an underlying hypothesis as to why this treatment should work?
> 3. Have trustworthy studies of efficacy been performed and published?
> 4. Do these studies come to a favorable conclusion regarding efficacy?
> 5. Does the risk/benefit ratio justify clinical use of the novel treatment?
>
> Many novel, alternative treatment options for AD are circulating on the Internet and in print media. Because there is no cure for AD, it is only logical that patients are interested in information on treatment of AD. Following the five simple questions of the Munich left hand rule regarding a new treatment helps clinicians and patients estimate the value of the new treatment and greatly reduce quackery in the field of AD therapy.

Clinical trial or in vitro data published for some other phytotherapeutics indicate a possible anti-inflammatory, antibacterial, or antipruritic effect suitable for AD treatment, but the evidence remains weak. Some of these phytotherapeutics contain essential oils, which are known contact allergens, especially when degrading after prolonged use or exposure to oxygen and light.[122–126] Use of phyotherapeutics should be evaluated carefully for the risk/benefit ratio.

ASSESSING PARAMEDICAL OR ALTERNATIVE TREATMENT SUGGESTIONS FOR AD

Because AD is a highly chronic skin disease without known cure but severely reduces the quality of life of affected patients, many patients with AD are interested in novel or paramedical treatment options for their disease. Every novel potential therapy for AD should be evaluated carefully for its efficacy and safety by the scientific community, keeping in mind that it is the duty of the manufacturer to provide this evidence. The Munich left hand rule for assessing new treatment of well-known diseases consists of five simple questions (**Box 2**) and is an easy procedure to delineate potentially useful novel treatment options from quackery or seemingly useful treatment suggestions that are not helpful in daily practice.

SUMMARY

Conventional therapy of AD has evolved and improved during the past decades. A better understanding of the impaired barrier function in AD and the mechanisms leading to increased susceptibility of patients with AD towards cutaneous infection will stimulate the development of better topical drugs, rebuilding the epidermal barrier and preventing microbial infection in patients with AD. The introduction of TCIs and, most recently, a proactive treatment approach have had an impact on the management of patients with AD and will hopefully lead to improvement in their quality of life. Ongoing and future research targeting the mechanisms of AD will eventually lead to even more promising treatment options.

REFERENCES

1. Schmid MH, Korting HC. Coal tar, pine tar and sulfonated shale oil preparations: comparative activity, efficacy and safety. Dermatology 1996;193(1):1–5.

2. Darsow U, Wollenberg A, Simon D, et al. ETFAD/EADV eczema task force 2009 position paper on diagnosis and treatment of atopic dermatitis. J Eur Acad Dermatol Venereol 2010;24(3):317–28.
3. Schmid-Grendelmeier P, Simon D, Simon HU, et al. Epidemiology, clinical features, and immunology of the "intrinsic" (non-IgE-mediated) type of atopic dermatitis (constitutional dermatitis). Allergy 2001;56(9):841–9.
4. Bieber T. Atopic dermatitis. N Engl J Med 2008;358(14):1483–94.
5. European Task Force on Atopic Dermatitis. Severity scoring of atopic dermatitis: the SCORAD Index. Dermatology 1993;186:23–31.
6. Elias PM, Hatano Y, Williams ML. Basis for the barrier abnormality in atopic dermatitis: outside-inside-outside pathogenic mechanisms. J Allergy Clin Immunol 2008;121(6):1337–43.
7. Cork MJ, Danby SG, Vasilopoulos Y, et al. Epidermal barrier dysfunction in atopic dermatitis. J Invest Dermatol 2009;129(8):1892–908.
8. Scott IR, Harding CR, Barrett JG. Histidine-rich protein of the keratohyalin granules. Source of the free amino acids, urocanic acid and pyrrolidone carboxylic acid in the stratum corneum. Biochim Biophys Acta 1982;719(1):110–7.
9. Meyer W, Poehling HM, Neurand K. Intraepidermal distribution of free amino acids in porcine skin. J Dermatol Sci 1991;2(5):383–92.
10. Smith FJ, Irvine AD, Terron-Kwiatkowski A, et al. Loss-of-function mutations in the gene encoding filaggrin cause ichthyosis vulgaris. Nat Genet 2006;38(3): 337–42.
11. Palmer CN, Irvine AD, Terron-Kwiatkowski A, et al. Common loss-of-function variants of the epidermal barrier protein filaggrin are a major predisposing factor for atopic dermatitis. Nat Genet 2006;38(4):441–6.
12. Weidinger S, Illig T, Baurecht H, et al. Loss-of-function variations within the filaggrin gene predispose for atopic dermatitis with allergic sensitizations. J Allergy Clin Immunol 2006;118(1):214–9.
13. Weidinger S, Rodriguez E, Stahl C, et al. Filaggrin mutations strongly predispose to early-onset and extrinsic atopic dermatitis. J Invest Dermatol 2007; 127(3):724–6.
14. Fallon PG, Sasaki T, Sandilands A, et al. A homozygous frameshift mutation in the mouse Flg gene facilitates enhanced percutaneous allergen priming. Nat Genet 2009;41(5):602–8.
15. Sandilands A, Sutherland C, Irvine AD, et al. Filaggrin in the frontline: role in skin barrier function and disease. J Cell Sci 2009;122(Pt 9):1285–94.
16. Williams HC. Evening primrose oil for atopic dermatitis. BMJ 2003;327(7428): 1358–9.
17. Sator PG, Schmidt JB, Honigsmann H. Comparison of epidermal hydration and skin surface lipids in healthy individuals and in patients with atopic dermatitis. J Am Acad Dermatol 2003;48(3):352–8.
18. Bleck O, Abeck D, Ring J, et al. Two ceramide subfractions detectable in Cer(AS) position by HPTLC in skin surface lipids of non-lesional skin of atopic eczema. J Invest Dermatol 1999;113(6):894–900.
19. Hara J, Higuchi K, Okamoto R, et al. High-expression of sphingomyelin deacylase is an important determinant of ceramide deficiency leading to barrier disruption in atopic dermatitis. J Invest Dermatol 2000;115(3):406–13.
20. Higuchi K, Hara J, Okamoto R, et al. The skin of atopic dermatitis patients contains a novel enzyme, glucosylceramide sphingomyelin deacylase, which cleaves the N-acyl linkage of sphingomyelin and glucosylceramide. Biochem J 2000;350(Pt 3):747–56.

21. Wollenberg A, Wetzel S, Burgdorf WHC, et al. Viral infections in atopic dermatitis: pathogenic aspects and clinical management. J Allergy Clin Immunol 2003;112:667–74.
22. Wollenberg A, Zoch C, Wetzel S, et al. Predisposing factors and clinical features of eczema herpeticum: a retrospective analysis of 100 cases. J Am Acad Dermatol 2003;49(2):198–205.
23. Mempel M, Lina G, Hojka M, et al. High prevalence of superantigens associated with the egc locus in *Staphylococcus aureus* isolates from patients with atopic eczema. Eur J Clin Microbiol Infect Dis 2003;22(5): 306–9.
24. Wollenberg A, Klein E. Current aspects of innate and adaptive immunity in atopic dermatitis. Clin Rev Allergy Immunol 2007;33(1–2):35–44.
25. Ong PY, Ohtake T, Brandt C, et al. Endogenous antimicrobial peptides and skin infections in atopic dermatitis. N Engl J Med 2002;347(15):1151–60.
26. Schauber J, Gallo RL. Antimicrobial peptides and the skin immune defense system. J Allergy Clin Immunol 2008;122(2):261–6.
27. Cho SH, Strickland I, Tomkinson A, et al. Preferential binding of *Staphylococcus aureus* to skin sites of Th2-mediated inflammation in a murine model. J Invest Dermatol 2001;116(5):658–63.
28. Mempel M, Schmidt T, Weidinger S, et al. Role of *Staphylococcus aureus* surface-associated proteins in the attachment to cultured HaCaT keratinocytes in a new adhesion assay. J Invest Dermatol 1998;111(3):452–6.
29. Kisich KO, Carspecken CW, Fieve S, et al. Defective killing of *Staphylococcus aureus* in atopic dermatitis is associated with reduced mobilization of human beta-defensin-3. J Allergy Clin Immunol 2008;122(1):62–8.
30. Mrabet-Dahbi S, Dalpke AH, Niebuhr M, et al. The Toll-like receptor 2 R753Q mutation modifies cytokine production and Toll-like receptor expression in atopic dermatitis. J Allergy Clin Immunol 2008;121(4):1013–9.
31. Bunikowski R, Mielke ME, Skarabis H, et al. Evidence for a disease-promoting effect of *Staphylococcus aureus*-derived exotoxins in atopic dermatitis. J Allergy Clin Immunol 2000;105(4):814–9.
32. Schnopp C, Grosch J, Ring J, et al. Microbial allergen-specific IgE is not suitable to identify the intrinsic form of atopic eczema in children. J Allergy Clin Immunol 2008;121(1):267–8, e261 [author reply: 268].
33. Mihm MC, Soter NA, Dvorak HF, et al. The structure of normal skin and the morphology of atopic eczema. J Invest Dermatol 1976;67:305–12.
34. Hanifin JM, Rajka G. Diagnostic features of atopic dermatitis. Acta Derm Venereol Suppl (Stockh) 1980;92:44–7.
35. Wollenberg A, Kraft S, Hanau D, et al. Immunomorphological and ultrastructural characterization of Langerhans cells and a novel, inflammatory dendritic epidermal cell (IDEC) population in lesional skin of atopic eczema. J Invest Dermatol 1996;106(3):446–53.
36. Maurer D, Fiebiger E, Ebner C, et al. Peripheral blood dendritic cells express FceRI as a complex composed of FceRIa and FceRIg-Chains and can use this Receptor for IgE-mediated Allergen presentation. J Immunol 1996;157: 607–16.
37. Sonkoly E, Muller A, Lauerma AI, et al. IL-31: a new link between T cells and pruritus in atopic skin inflammation. J Allergy Clin Immunol 2006;117(2): 411–7.
38. Wollenberg A, Bieber T. Proactive therapy of atopic dermatitis—an emerging concept. Allergy 2009;64:276–8.

39. Wollenberg A, Frank R, Kroth J, et al. Proactive therapy of atopic eczema—an evidence-based concept with a behavioral background. J Dtsch Dermatol Ges 2009;7:117–21.

40. Buraczewska I, Berne B, Lindberg M, et al. Changes in skin barrier function following long-term treatment with moisturizers, a randomized controlled trial. Br J Dermatol 2007;156(3):492–8.

41. Wohlrab J. Adjuvante Therapie der atopischen Dermatitis. Vol. 5, 2005.

42. Gehring W. Basic therapy in atopic eczema. In: Ring J, Przybilla B, Ruzicka T, editors. Handbook or atopic eczema. 2nd edition. Berlin: Springer; 2005. p. 453–67.

43. Akdis CA, Akdis M, Bieber T, et al. Diagnosis and treatment of atopic dermatitis in children and adults: European Academy of Allergology and Clinical Immunology/American Academy of Allergy, Asthma and Immunology/PRACTALL Consensus Report. Allergy 2006;61(8):969–87.

44. Elias PM. An appropriate response to the black-box warning: corrective, barrier repair therapy in atopic dermatitis. Clin Med Dermatol 2009;2:1–3.

45. Szczepanowska J, Reich A, Szepietowski JC. Emollients improve treatment results with topical corticosteroids in childhood atopic dermatitis: a randomized comparative study. Pediatr Allergy Immunol 2008;19(7):614–8.

46. Cork MJ, Britton J, Butler L, et al. Comparison of parent knowledge, therapy utilization and severity of atopic eczema before and after explanation and demonstration of topical therapies by a specialist dermatology nurse. Br J Dermatol 2003;149(3):582–9.

47. Eberlein B, Eicke C, Reinhardt HW, et al. Adjuvant treatment of atopic eczema: assessment of an emollient containing N-palmitoylethanolamine (ATOPA study). J Eur Acad Dermatol Venereol 2008;22(1):73–82.

48. Sugarman JL, Parish LC. Efficacy of a lipid-based barrier repair formulation in moderate-to-severe pediatric atopic dermatitis. J Drugs Dermatol 2009;8(12): 1106–11.

49. Jensen JM, Pfeiffer S, Witt M, et al. Different effects of pimecrolimus and betamethasone on the skin barrier in patients with atopic dermatitis. J Allergy Clin Immunol 2009;124(3 Suppl 2):R19–28.

50. Kao JS, Fluhr JW, Man MQ, et al. Short-term glucocorticoid treatment compromises both permeability barrier homeostasis and stratum corneum integrity: inhibition of epidermal lipid synthesis accounts for functional abnormalities. J Invest Dermatol 2003;120(3):456–64.

51. Leyden JJ, Marples RR, Kligman AM. Staphylococcus aureus in the lesions of atopic dermatitis. Br J Dermatol 1974;90(5):525–30.

52. Aly R, Maibach HI, Shinefield HR. Microbial flora of atopic dermatitis. Arch Dermatol 1977;113(6):780–2.

53. Breuer K, Haussler S, Kapp A, et al. Staphylococcus aureus: colonizing features and influence of an antibacterial treatment in adults with atopic dermatitis. Br J Dermatol 2002;147(1):55–61.

54. Hoeger PH, Lenz W, Boutonnier A, et al. Staphylococcal skin colonization in children with atopic dermatitis: prevalence, persistence, and transmission of toxigenic and nontoxigenic strains. J Infect Dis 1992;165(6):1064–8.

55. Ewing CI, Ashcroft C, Gibbs AC, et al. Flucloxacillin in the treatment of atopic dermatitis. Br J Dermatol 1998;138(6):1022–9.

56. Hayakawa K, Hirahara K, Fukuda T, et al. Risk factors for severe impetiginized atopic dermatitis in Japan and assessment of its microbiological features. Clin Exp Dermatol 2009;34(5):e63–5.

57. Stalder JF, Fleury M, Sourisse M, et al. Local steroid therapy and bacterial skin flora in atopic dermatitis. Br J Dermatol 1994;131(4):536–40.
58. Remitz A, Kyllonen H, Granlund H, et al. Tacrolimus ointment reduces staphylococcal colonization of atopic dermatitis lesions. J Allergy Clin Immunol 2001; 107:196–7.
59. Boguniewicz M, Leung DY. Pathophysiologic mechanisms in atopic dermatitis. Semin Cutan Med Surg 2001;20(4):217–25.
60. Birnie AJ, Bath-Hextall FJ, Ravenscroft JC, et al. Interventions to reduce Staphylococcus aureus in the management of atopic eczema. Cochrane Database Syst Rev 2008;(3):CD003871.
61. Lever R, Hadley K, Downey D, et al. Staphylococcal colonization in atopic dermatitis and the effect of topical mupirocin therapy. Br J Dermatol 1988; 119(2):189–98.
62. Gong JQ, Lin L, Lin T, et al. Skin colonization by Staphylococcus aureus in patients with eczema and atopic dermatitis and relevant combined topical therapy: a double-blind multicentre randomized controlled trial. Br J Dermatol 2006;155(4):680–7.
63. Schuttelaar ML, Coenraads PJ. A randomized, double-blind study to assess the efficacy of addition of tetracycline to triamcinolone acetonide in the treatment of moderate to severe atopic dermatitis. J Eur Acad Dermatol Venereol 2008;22(9): 1076–82.
64. Yang LP, Keam SJ. Retapamulin: a review of its use in the management of impetigo and other uncomplicated superficial skin infections. Drugs 2008;68(6): 855–73.
65. Gloor M, Becker A, Wasik B, et al. [Triclosan, a topical dermatologic agent. In vitro- and in vivo studies on the effectiveness of a new preparation in the New German Formulary]. Hautarzt 2002;53(11):724–9 [in German].
66. Ledder RG, Gilbert P, Willis C, et al. Effects of chronic triclosan exposure upon the antimicrobial susceptibility of 40 ex-situ environmental and human isolates. J Appl Microbiol 2006;100(5):1132–40.
67. Moss T, Howes D, Williams FM. Percutaneous penetration and dermal metabolism of triclosan (2,4, 4'-trichloro-2'-hydroxydiphenyl ether). Food Chem Toxicol 2000;38(4):361–70.
68. Allmyr M, Adolfsson-Erici M, McLachlan MS, et al. Triclosan in plasma and milk from Swedish nursing mothers and their exposure via personal care products. Sci Total Environ 2006;372(1):87–93.
69. Dayan AD. Risk assessment of triclosan [Irgasan] in human breast milk. Food Chem Toxicol 2007;45(1):125–9.
70. Tan WP, Suresh S, Tey HL, et al. A randomized double-blind controlled trial to compare a triclosan-containing emollient with vehicle for the treatment of atopic dermatitis. Clin Exp Dermatol 2010;35(4):e109–12.
71. Stalder JF, Fleury M, Sourisse M, et al. Comparative effects of two topical antiseptics (chlorhexidine vs KMnO4) on bacterial skin flora in atopic dermatitis. Acta Derm Venereol Suppl (Stockh) 1992;176:132–4.
72. Jee R, Nel L, Gnanakumaran G, et al. Four cases of anaphylaxis to chlorhexidine impregnated central venous catheters: a case cluster or the tip of the iceberg? Br J Anaesth 2009;103(4):614–5.
73. Nagendran V, Wicking J, Ekbote A, et al. IgE-mediated chlorhexidine allergy: a new occupational hazard? Occup Med (Lond) 2009;59(4):270–2.
74. Garvey LH, Kroigaard M, Poulsen LK, et al. IgE-mediated allergy to chlorhexidine. J Allergy Clin Immunol 2007;120(2):409–15.

75. Huang JT, Abrams M, Tlougan B, et al. Treatment of *Staphylococcus aureus* colonization in atopic dermatitis decreases disease severity. Pediatrics 2009; 123(5):e808–14.
76. Sugimoto K, Ishikawa N, Terano T, et al. The importance of bacterial superantigens produced by *Staphylococcus aureus* in the treatment of atopic dermatitis using povidone-iodine. Dermatology 2006;212(Suppl 1):26–34.
77. Sugimoto K, Kuroki H, Kanazawa M, et al. New successful treatment with disinfectant for atopic dermatitis. Dermatology 1997;195(Suppl 2):62–8.
78. Akiyama H, Tada J, Toi J, et al. Changes in *Staphylococcus aureus* density and lesion severity after topical application of povidone-iodine in cases of atopic dermatitis. J Dermatol Sci 1997;16(1):23–30.
79. Gauger A, Fischer S, Mempel M, et al. Efficacy and functionality of silver-coated textiles in patients with atopic eczema. J Eur Acad Dermatol Venereol 2006; 20(5):534–41.
80. Koller DY, Halmerbauer G, Bock A, et al. Action of a silk fabric treated with AEGIS in children with atopic dermatitis: a 3-month trial. Pediatr Allergy Immunol 2007;18(4):335–8.
81. Stinco G, Piccirillo F, Valent F. A randomized double-blind study to investigate the clinical efficacy of adding a non-migrating antimicrobial to a special silk fabric in the treatment of atopic dermatitis. Dermatology 2008;217(3):191–5.
82. Darsow U, Lubbe J, Taieb A, et al. Position paper on diagnosis and treatment of atopic dermatitis. J Eur Acad Dermatol Venereol 2005;19(3):286–95.
83. Walsh P, Aeling JL, Huff L, et al. Hypothalamus-pituitary-adrenal axis suppression by superpotent topical steroids. J Am Acad Dermatol 1993; 29(3):501–3.
84. Charman C, Williams H. The use of corticosteroids and corticosteroid phobia in atopic dermatitis. Clin Dermatol 2003;21(3):193–200.
85. Zuberbier T, Orlow SJ, Paller AS, et al. Patient perspectives on the management of atopic dermatitis. J Allergy Clin Immunol 2006;118(1):226–32.
86. Bornhövd E, Burgdorf WHC, Wollenberg A. Macrolactam immunomodulators for topical treatment of inflammatory skin diseases. J Am Acad Dermatol 2001;45: 736–43.
87. Ruzicka T, Bieber T, Schöpf E, et al. A short-term trial of tacrolimus ointment for atopic dermatitis. N Engl J Med 1997;337:816–21.
88. Van Leent EJ, Graber M, Thurston M, et al. Effectiveness of the ascomycin macrolactam SDZ ASM 981 in the topical treatment of atopic dermatitis. Arch Dermatol 1998;134(7):805–9.
89. Reitamo S, Rustin M, Ruzicka T, et al. Efficacy and safety of tacrolimus ointment compared with that of hydrocortisone butyrate ointment in adult patients with atopic dermatitis. J Allergy Clin Immunol 2002;109:547–55.
90. Luger T, Van-Leent EJ, Graeber M, et al. SDZ ASM 981: an emerging safe and effective treatment for atopic dermatitis. Br J Dermatol 2001;144(4):788–94.
91. Ring J, Barker J, Behrendt H, et al. Review of the potential photococarcinogenicity of topical calcineurin inhibitors: position statement of the European Dermatology Forum. J Eur Acad Dermatol Venereol 2005;19(6): 663–71.
92. Wollenberg A, Reitamo S, Girolomoni G, et al. Proactive treatment of atopic dermatitis in adults with 0.1% tacrolimus ointment. Allergy 2008;63(7):742–50.
93. Lübbe J, Pournaras CC, Saurat JH. Eczema herpeticum during treatment of atopic dermatitis with 0.1% tacrolimus ointment. Dermatology 2000;201(3): 249–51.

94. Wetzel S, Wollenberg A. Eczema molluscatum in tacrolimus treated atopic dermatitis. Eur J Dermatol 2004;14(1):73–4.
95. Reitamo S, Rissanen J, Remitz A, et al. Tacrolimus ointment does not affect collagen synthesis: results of a single-center randomized trial. J Invest Dermatol 1998;111:396–8.
96. Queille-Roussel C, Paul C, Duteil L, et al. The new topical ascomycin derivative SDZ ASM 981 does not induce skin atrophy when applied to normal skin for 4 weeks: a randomized, double-blind controlled study. Br J Dermatol 2001;144:507–13.
97. Arellano FM, Wentworth CE, Arana A, et al. Risk of lymphoma following exposure to calcineurin inhibitors and topical steroids in patients with atopic dermatitis. J Invest Dermatol 2007;127(4):808–16.
98. Margolis DJ, Hoffstad O, Bilker W. Lack of association between exposure to topical calcineurin inhibitors and skin cancer in adults. Dermatology 2007;214(4):289–95.
99. Reitamo S, Wollenberg A, Schopf E, et al. Safety and efficacy of 1 year of tacrolimus ointment monotherapy in adults with atopic dermatitis. The European Tacrolimus Ointment Study Group. Arch Dermatol 2000;136(8):999–1006.
100. Thaci D, Reitamo S, Gonzalez Ensenat MA, et al. Proactive disease management with 0.03% tacrolimus ointment for children with atopic dermatitis: results of a randomized, multicentre, comparative study. Br J Dermatol 2008;159(6):1348–56.
101. Hoeger PH, Lee KH, Jautova J, et al. The treatment of facial atopic dermatitis in children who are intolerant of, or dependent on, topical corticosteroids: a randomized, controlled clinical trial. Br J Dermatol 2009;160(2):415–22.
102. Wollenberg A, Reitamo S, Atzori F, et al. Proactive treatment of atopic dermatitis in adults with 0.1% tacrolimus ointment. Allergy 2008;63(6):742–50.
103. Proksch E, Folster-Holst R, Jensen JM. Skin barrier function, epidermal proliferation and differentiation in eczema. J Dermatol Sci 2006;43(3):159–69.
104. Kerschenlohr K, Darsow U, Burgdorf WH, et al. Lessons from atopy patch testing in atopic dermatitis. Curr Allergy Asthma Rep 2004;4(4):285–9.
105. Darsow U, Laifaoui J, Kerschenlohr K, et al. The prevalence of positive reactions in the atopy patch test with aeroallergens and food allergens in subjects with atopic eczema: a European multicenter study. Allergy 2004;59(12):1318–25.
106. Macheleidt O, Kaiser HW, Sandhoff K. Deficiency of epidermal protein-bound omega-hydroxyceramides in atopic dermatitis. J Invest Dermatol 2002;119(1):166–73.
107. Howell MD, Kim BE, Gao P, et al. Cytokine modulation of atopic dermatitis filaggrin skin expression. J Allergy Clin Immunol 2007;120(1):150–5.
108. Bieber T, Braun-Falco O. IgE-bearing Langerhans cells are not specific to atopic eczema but are found in inflammatory skin diseases. J Am Acad Dermatol 1991;24(4):658–9.
109. Bieber T, de la Salle H, Wollenberg A, et al. Human epidermal Langerhans cells express the high affinity receptor for immunoglobulin E (Fc epsilon RI). J Exp Med 1992;175(5):1285–90.
110. Wang B, Rieger A, Kilgus O, et al. Epidermal Langerhans cells from normal human skin bind monomeric IgE via FceRI. J Exp Med 1992;175:1353–65.
111. Semper AE, Heron K, Woollard AC, et al. Surface expression of Fc epsilon RI on Langerhans' cells of clinically uninvolved skin is associated with disease activity in atopic dermatitis, allergic asthma, and rhinitis. J Allergy Clin Immunol 2003;112(2):411–9.

112. Wollenberg A, Wen S, Bieber T. Phenotyping of epidermal dendritic cells: clinical applications of a flow cytometric micromethod. Cytometry 1999;37:147–55.
113. Wollenberg A, Sidhu MK, Odeyemi I, et al. Economic evaluation of maintenance treatment with tacrolimus 0.1% ointment in adults with moderate to severe atopic dermatitis. Br J Dermatol 2008;159(6):1322–30.
114. Breneman D, Fleischer AB Jr, Abramovits W, et al. Intermittent therapy for flare prevention and long-term disease control in stabilized atopic dermatitis: a randomized comparison of 3-times-weekly applications of tacrolimus ointment versus vehicle. J Am Acad Dermatol 2008;58(6):990–9.
115. Hanifin J, Gupta AK, Rajagopalan R. Intermittent dosing of fluticasone propionate cream for reducing the risk of relapse in atopic dermatitis patients. Br J Dermatol 2002;147(3):528–37.
116. Berth-Jones J, Damstra RJ, Golsch S, et al. Twice weekly fluticasone propionate added to emollient maintenance treatment to reduce risk of relapse in atopic dermatitis: randomised, double blind, parallel group study. BMJ 2003; 326(7403):1367–72.
117. Peserico A, Stadtler G, Sebastian M, et al. Reduction of relapses of atopic dermatitis with methylprednisolone aceponate cream twice weekly in addition to maintenance treatment with emollient: a multicentre, randomized, double-blind, controlled study. Br J Dermatol 2008;158(4):801–7.
118. Heine G, Schnuch A, Uter W, et al. Type-IV sensitization profile of individuals with atopic eczema: results from the Information Network of Departments of Dermatology (IVDK) and the German Contact Dermatitis Research Group (DKG). Allergy 2006;61(5):611–6.
119. Heine G, Schnuch A, Uter W, et al. Frequency of contact allergy in German children and adolescents patch tested between 1995 and 2002: results from the Information Network of Departments of Dermatology and the German Contact Dermatitis Research Group. Contact Derm 2004;51(3):111–7.
120. Schempp CM, Hezel S, Simon JC. [Topical treatment of atopic dermatitis with Hypericum cream. A randomised, placebo-controlled, double-blind half-side comparison study]. Hautarzt Mar 2003;54(3):248–53 [in German].
121. Hoare C, Li Wan Po A, Williams H. Systematic review of treatments for atopic eczema. Health Technol Assess 2000;4(37):1–191.
122. Hagvall L, Skold M, Brared-Christensson J, et al. Lavender oil lacks natural protection against autoxidation, forming strong contact allergens on air exposure. Contact Derm 2008;59(3):143–50.
123. Adisen E, Onder M. Allergic contact dermatitis from Laurus nobilis oil induced by massage. Contact Derm 2007;56(6):360–1.
124. Rutherford T, Nixon R, Tam M, et al. Allergy to tea tree oil: retrospective review of 41 cases with positive patch tests over 4.5 years. Australas J Dermatol 2007; 48(2):83–7.
125. Corazza M, Lauriola MM, Poli F, et al. Contact vulvitis due to Pseudowintera Colorata in a topical herbal medicament. Acta Derm Venereol 2007;87(2):178–9.
126. Simpson EL, Law SV, Storrs FJ. Prevalence of botanical extract allergy in patients with contact dermatitis. Dermatitis 2004;15(2):67–72.

The Role of the Nurse Educator in Managing Atopic Dermatitis

Noreen Heer Nicol, MS, RN, FNP[a,b,c,]*,
Steven J. Ersser, PhD (Lond), RN, CertTHEd[c,d]

KEYWORDS

• Nurse educator • Patient education • Atopic dermatitis
• Atopic eczema

Atopic dermatitis (AD), also known as atopic eczema, is the most common chronic, relapsing skin disorder seen in infants and children, although it can affect patients of any age. The prevalence of AD has increased globally, with more than half of these patients developing asthma and allergies.[1,2] A significant economic burden on the patient, family, and society is experienced because of AD.[3,4] Successful conventional strategies for managing AD require an accurate diagnosis, identification, and elimination of exacerbating factors including irritants and allergens, adequate hydration of the skin, control of pruritus and infections, and appropriate use of topical anti-inflammatory and other medications.[5,6] Appropriate and effective AD management requires that health care professionals become increasingly aware of the social context of the disease and the effect on the lives of those affected.[7] Successful strategies, particularly in those patients with moderate-to-severe disease, have been influenced by the commitment and expertise of the multidisciplinary approach led by physicians and nurses in the past 2 decades.[8,9] Educational interventions have long been recommended and used as a critical adjunct at all levels of therapy for patients with AD to enhance therapy effectiveness. By using education to enhance the effectiveness of treatment, health care professionals can affect quality of life in a significant manner.[10]

[a] Professional Development, The Children's Hospital, Denver, CO, USA
[b] University of Colorado - Clinical Sciences, Denver, CO, USA
[c] Nursing Advisory Board, International Skin Care Nursing Group, London WC2H 9NS, UK
[d] Centre for Wellbeing & Quality of Life, School of Health & Social Care, Bournemouth University, Bournemouth BH1 3LT, UK
* Corresponding author. Professional Development, The Children's Hospital, National Jewish Health, Denver, CO.
E-mail address: nicol.noreen@tchden.org

Immunol Allergy Clin N Am 30 (2010) 369–383
doi:10.1016/j.iac.2010.06.007
0889-8561/10/$ – see front matter © 2010 Published by Elsevier Inc.
immunology.theclinics.com

GOALS OF EDUCATION

Experts from the European Academy of Allergy and Clinical Immunology and the American Academy of Allergy, Asthma and Immunology developed consensus guidelines for AD in the Practical Allergy (PRACTALL) initiative.[11] They stated that the goal of patient education should be living with AD by means of an empowered patient or, in the case of infants and young children, a caregiver who can work as a partner with the doctor, or health care team, in self-managing their own or their children's disease. A critical objective is to enable patients to be as effective as possible in helping themselves and engaging in effective self-management.[12] Other educational goals or outcomes include reduction of doctor shopping, facilitating a more effective partnership between the health care provider and patient-parent, and decreasing the long-term costs of chronic disease treatment.

Structured patient education should enable both the patient and the parent to have realistic short-term goals, enter a process of problem solving, accept living with disease, ensure the appropriate use of available social support, and enhance the motivation for therapy. These interventions may be directed toward adult patients, parents, or children with eczema, with parents often the primary focus of such educational approaches.

Education may need to extend to other family members, caregivers, school staff, and to the work environment to ensure its effectiveness. The educational content must include teaching about the chronic or relapsing nature of AD, exacerbating factors, and therapeutic options that are important to both patients and caregivers.[13] Important educational goals are becoming increasingly difficult to accomplish in the current health care environment and seem equally difficult to measure; these issues are highlighted in this article. The current lack of adequate trial evidence of the effectiveness of educational interventions in the care of AD are also addressed. This review focuses on the most common educational interventions being used today internationally in the care of patients with AD.

EDUCATION STRATEGIES

Educational strategies are focused on the process of gaining new knowledge and/or skills through teaching and learning activities. The approach involves information giving and formal teaching to help recipients become more accurately informed about their condition and more knowledgeable and skilful in managing their illness. This information should better equip them to understand the need for medical treatments and disease prevention. Educational interventions may include various learning tools including lectures, audiotapes, books, booklets, leaflets, handouts, films, videotapes, computer-assisted instruction, home care plans, or action plans. The content of these educational interventions may include information on the disease, treatment instructions, prevention, and management strategies. They may be delivered through one-on-one communication, direct demonstration with reinforcement, role playing, group discussions with question-and-answer sessions, classroom teaching in the hospital or clinic setting, or in the community via an outreach program mediated through the home or school.

THE EDUCATION TEAM

Almost universally, eczema education is increasingly difficult to accomplish in the typical AD clinic visit. Adequate time is needed to discuss this chronic illness, potential triggers, and diagnostic and treatment options, irrespective of degree of disease severity.[14,15] The time that patients and families spend at an initial visit and follow-up visits varies greatly across specialties and across the world. Regardless of the severity of the disease, a new patient visit can be as short as 5 minutes or as long as 90 to 120 minutes. The follow-up visits are usually considerably less. These resource-related time pressures have implications for the effectiveness of educational opportunities. Which, or how many, different health care professionals deliver the components of care and education varies almost as much as the length of time spent with the patient and family. The range of professional delivery is diverse, including a single physician, physician and registered or specialist nurse team, a nurse-led clinic, or a large multidisciplinary team. One recent review using a multidisciplinary approach involved a team composed of pediatric allergist-immunologists with extensive experience in basic and clinical research in AD, a nurse practitioner/dermatology clinical specialist, pediatric psychiatrist, psychosocial clinicians, allergy-immunology fellows-in-training, physician assistants, nurse educators, child life specialists, dieticians, and rehabilitation therapists.[8]

MODELS OF DELIVERY

Nurse-led approaches have been the subject of a comprehensive Cochrane review.[16] This systematic review of educational interventions for managing AD in children, revealed 2 key models of delivery in Europe. Such interventions have been used as an adjunct to conventional therapy to enhance the effectiveness of topical therapy. One model was nurse-led practice in which nurses delivered education systematically to the parent and child, reflecting common practice in the United Kingdom and other parts of Europe. Other areas have used a multidisciplinary approach, but one that is different to that described earlier. An additional key model is the eczema school, also used primarily in Europe, involving a more extensive and prolonged educational program delivered by a multiprofessional health team.

Although AD patients of all severities benefit from a comprehensive management approach that incorporates education, only a subset of patients receive in-depth education, in accordance with the organization of service delivery. These patients tend to include those who are failing conventional therapy, those with concerns about medication side effects, those whose disease is causing a significant effect on their and their family's quality of life, and those with recurrent skin infections or on frequent courses of antibiotics. These groups are all candidates for a comprehensive approach to management that highlights education.

The patient and family with chronic AD have often seen multiple health care providers who may have given them confusing or conflicting information. This experience may set up a cycle of frustration and search for a straightforward solution to their problem. Practitioners of unproven therapies may take advantage of these patients, even promising a cure.[17] Thus, it becomes imperative to convey the message that, at present, treatment is directed at levels of control, not a cure. However, in the patient with severe, difficult-to-control disease, education is an especially critical part of illness management. This issue also highlights the crucial need for a consistent educational message to avoid confusion and, as such, there is significant value when 1 member of the team provides this education, but does so within a team context with case liaison. In a related way, the eczema school model would need to operate toward a curriculum that provides for the continuity and coherence of the approach required from the team.

Another teaching strategy includes group instruction, including the eczema school model, highlighted earlier. Smaller-scale hospital programs have been established in some centers.[18] In the United States, Nicol and Boguniewicz[5] described a hospital-based program including a weekly 1-hour class addressing various aspects of AD. This class is taught by dedicated registered nurses to supplement teaching that occurs in the clinic, day program, or inpatient settings. Content of the slide lecture reflects input from the multidisciplinary team and is routinely reviewed and updated. The long-term success of this intervention has not been systematically evaluated but is likely to be related to the competency and consistency of the staff providing these lectures or group activities.

A Cochrane review of educational interventions for atopic eczema[16] studied the contrasting nurse-led versus eczema school models of educational delivery. A small number of studies met the methodological quality threshold for inclusion within the review. Four studies related to educational intervention met the inclusion criteria.[19–22] Two[19,20] studies describe the eczema school model and 2[21,22] studies evaluated nurse-led education. The 4 studies focused on intervention that was directed toward the parents, although the outcome measures included largely child-related outcomes.

Data synthesis was not possible because of the heterogeneity of the data, and especially the various outcome measures adopted. However, some individual rigorous educational studies identified significant improvements in disease severity between intervention groups. These studies included the large German trial by Staab and colleagues[20] of 820 children, which evaluated long-term outcomes and found significant improvements in both disease severity at 3 months to 7 years, $(P = .0002)$, 8 to 12 years, $(P = .003)$, 13 to 18 years, $(P = .0001)$, and parental quality of life at 3 months to 7 years, $(P = .0001)$, 8 to 12 years, $(P = .002)$, for children with atopic eczema. However, this intervention seems to be resource intensive compared with the nurse-led models. Niebel and colleagues[21] found video-based education more effective in improving severity than direct education and the control $(P<.001)$, highlighting the need to consider technologically supported learning approaches. Nurse-led education and support-focused clinics have also been established for adults in dermatology, and a few have been evaluated,[23] although additional evidence of their effect on eczema populations is required. These nurse-led approaches provide considerable scope for nursing staff to approach the assessment and management of educational and support needs in a systematic way and thereby enable more evaluations of their relative effectiveness.

In principle, the nurse-led consultation model provides an opportunity to target educational needs to ensure that treatment failure caused by poor adherence is less likely; this also permits the physician more time to focus on diagnostic and related treatment issues. Treatment adherence remains a key issue for managing AD.[18] Nurses can play a key role in improving adherence within the dermatology field by providing systematic education to patients to achieve the necessary degree of behavioral change needed to manage chronic interventions.[24] The effect of these areas requires further research evaluation. To use time effectively for both the patient and family and clinical staff, such clinics may need to be organized in sequence with overlap between the patient seeing the physician and the nurse to aid effective communication and continuity.

Examining the European nurse-led model within the United States context, the time that nurses spend educating AD patients in the United States is largely viewed as a free and nonreimbursable activity that is unlike the European model, which embraces the nurse-led management and education role. The fee-for-service billing system related to AD care in the United States has never promoted, nor been able to reimburse, the nurse education models as they have for some other chronic diseases, such as diabetes. The differences between the United States and European models have been a barrier to studying and promoting a common benchmark of optimal-practice nursing education.

A considerable number of issues remain, including the development of optimal timing of therapeutically effective and resource—efficient consultations, the frequency and duration of support, and whether learning is more effective when undertaken in a single session with follow-up telephone consultation.

AD SELF-MANAGEMENT PLANS AND WRITTEN INSTRUCTIONS

There are many ways to customize care plans to meet the needs of patient's and families. Development of a skin care regimen that is agreed on by the clinician, patient, or caregivers requires open communication. Patients and caregivers may forget or confuse skin care recommendations given to them without a written plan. The significant sleep deprivation and disturbances that accompany chronic AD make this confusion more likely. Such approaches help the nurse target the specific skills or knowledge that enable more effective self-management. This plan may specify learning objectives and allow for review and modification as required at follow-up visits.

A multidisciplinary care approach used for the past 2 decades at one tertiary care center includes education using a stepwise approach, allowing the patient to decrease or increase treatment for AD, as warranted by AD severity.[8] The program has been providing participants and families with a detailed, written home step-care plan for more than 20 years. Historically, these individualized care plans were extremely labor intensive and included a personalized booklet with annotated photographs reflecting stages of disease specific to that patient and remission with appropriate skin care.[5] The current home care plans continue to be individualized but follow a more standardized format and address treatment in a step-care manner (**Box 1**).

The approach confirms the importance of teaching patients skills to self-monitor and manage diseases and to use a written home care plan, referred to as the AD action plan. The action plan used for AD has similarities with the more recent asthma action plan, and many patients have both conditions. The 2007 National Asthma Education and Prevention Program: Expert Panel Report 3 (EPR-3) confirms the importance of teaching patients skills to self-monitor and manage asthma and to use a written asthma action plan that should include instructions for daily treatment and ways to recognize and handle worsening disease.[25] The EPR-3 emphasizes the use of a stepwise approach in dealing with chronic inflammatory disease. This treatment model requires that all members of the multidisciplinary team teach the same key concepts and reinforce the messages being delivered to the patients and caregivers regardless of which educational strategy is incorporated. A recent small study of pediatricians and pediatric dermatologists in the United States showed that pediatricians are open to using AD action plans.[26]

AD EDUCATION TOPICS

The importance of education as a basis for improving adherence to treatment is highlighted in the United Kingdom's National Institute for Health and Clinical Excellence[27] evidence-based guidance on atopic eczema in children. It highlights the importance of educating both child and parent or caregiver with reinforcement at every consultation, both in written and verbal forms, with practical demonstrations covering how much treatment to use, how often to apply treatments, when and how to increase or decrease treatments, and how to treat infected AD.

Box 1

National Jewish Atopic Dermatitis Program step-care AD action plan

Take action with daily soak-and-seal skin care

MAINTENANCE OR DAILY CARE
Take at least one bath or shower per day; use warm water, for 10-15 minutes.
Use a gentle cleansing bar or wash in the sensitive skin formulation as needed such as Dove® or Oil of Olay®.
Pat away excess water and immediately (within 3 minutes) apply moisturizer, sealer, or maintenance medication if directed. Fragrance-free moisturizers available in one pound jars include Aquaphor® Ointment, Eucerin® Crème, Vanicream®, CeraVe® Cream or Cetaphil® Cream. Vaseline® is a good occlusive preparation to seal in the water; however, it contains no water so it only works effectively after a bathing. Use moisturizers liberally throughout the day. Moisturizers and sealers should not be applied over any topical medication.
Avoid skin irritants and proven allergens.

NOTES :
_____

_____

MILD TO MODERATE ATOPIC DERMATITIS
Bathe as above for 10-15 minutes, once (and possibly twice) daily.
Use cleansers as above.
Use moisturizers as above to healed and unaffected skin, twice daily especially after baths and at mid-day total body.
Apply to affected areas of face, groin and underarms twice daily especially after baths _____(low potency topical corticosteroid), or_____ (topical calcineurin inhibitors), or other topical preparation as directed _____ (topical barrier repair cream, eg. Atopiclair® three times daily).
Apply to other affected areas of the body twice daily especially after baths _____(low to mid- potency topical corticosteroid), or _____(topical calcineurin inhibitors), or other topical preparation as directed _____.

NOTES :
_____

_____

MODERATE TO SEVERE ATOPIC DERMATITIS
Bathe as above for 10-15 minutes, two times a day, once before bedtime.
Use cleansers as above or consider an antibacterial cleanser (eg. Lever 2000®)
Use moisturizers as above to healed and unaffected skin, twice daily especially after baths and at mid-day total body.
Apply to affected areas of face, groin and underarms twice daily especially after baths _____(low potency topical corticosteroid), or_____ (topical calcineurin inhibitors), or other topical preparation as directed _____ (topical barrier repair cream, eg. Atopiclair® three times daily).
Apply to other affected areas of the body twice daily especially after baths _____(mid- to high- potency topical corticosteroid), or _____ topical calcineurin inhibitors), or other topical preparation as directed.
Use wet wraps to involved areas selectively as directed.
Add other medications as directed: _____(eg. oral sedating antihistamines, topical or oral antimicrobial therapy)
Pay close attention to things that seem to irritate the skin or make condition worse.
Contact your health care provider for additional evaluation or therapies. Oral steroids are not usually recommended.
Step down to moderate plan above as the skin heals.

NOTES :
_____

_____

Reduce Skin Irritation
Wash all new clothes before wearing them. This removes formaldehyde and other irritating chemicals.
Add a second rinse cycle to ensure removal of detergent. Residual laundry detergent, particularly perfume or dye, may be irritating when it remains in the clothing. Changing to a liquid and fragrance-free, dye-free detergent may be helpful.
Wear garments that allow air to pass freely to your skin. Open weave, loose-fitting, cotton-blend clothing may be most comfortable.
Work and sleep in comfortable surroundings with a fairly constant temperature and humidity level.
Keep fingernails very short and smooth to help prevent damage due to scratching.
Carry a small tube of moisturizer/sunscreen at all times. Day-care/school/work should have a separate supply of moisturizer.
Shower or bathe after swimming in chlorinated pool or using hot tub using a gentle cleanser to remove chemicals, then apply moisturizer.

Developed by Noreen Nicol, RN, MS, FNP, Mark Boguniewicz, MD, Donald Leung, MD, PhD; Atopic Dermatitis Program, National Jewish Health, Denver, Colorado. Updated 2008. This may be modified and used for patient care citing National Jewish Health Atopic Dermatitis Program as source.

Such interventions may be illustrated with appropriate hands-on demonstrations. The suitability of such interventions depends on the age and developmental stage of the child.

The teaching about topical medications encompasses all the important dimensions of how, what, where, when, and why. The "how" is the need to ensure appropriate use.

Direct demonstration of effective skin care includes topical application of agents and techniques such as wet-wrap therapy.[5,6,28,29] Although modeling of the technique allows for vicarious experience to be gained, this should be followed up with observed practice by the practitioner, to enable confidence and performance accomplishment to be achieved. Such strategies help to build self-efficacy; that is, a person's or care giver's belief in their capacity to engage in specific health behavior such as eczema care, and is more likely to result in successful outcomes.[30] Watching the patient's or caregiver's current technique often reveals fundamental errors that may give providers valuable insights into why a patient may not be showing the expected therapeutic response. A typical example is that of the patient who was observed to apply a minute quantity of medication from a small tube over a large area. On examination of the dispensed medication, the tube, which should have lasted for only 2 weeks, still remained partially full after 3 months. This educational interaction provides a teaching opportunity to discuss risks or benefits of specific treatments, appropriate amounts to dispense and use, and other practical points.

Appropriate quantities of topical medications to apply are often most usefully communicated by helping patients and caregivers to understand the proportions of a tub or tube of medication to be used either per application or per day, or related practical measures such as a tablespoonful. These concepts are often easier to understand than measures such as fingertip units (FTU), where 1 FTU is approximately 500 mg. This amount of medication is expressed from a tube with a standard 5-mm diameter nozzle, applied from the distal crease to the tip of the index finger.[31] Such measures can be useful conceptually for health professionals, but the quantities involved can be impractical when considering the amount of emollient needed for therapeutic effectiveness. If the discussion is complicated by using a medication on affected areas and a moisturizer on nonaffected areas, one needs to be certain that the patient or caregiver understands the difference and which medication goes where.

Demonstrations can also be useful for group education, because they ensure that time is used effectively, as long as individual needs are addressed. If the educational group involves patients or parental caregivers with experience and skill in using eczema care techniques, such social learning can help to reinforce key messages, skills, and effectiveness. These approaches are also consistent with Bandura's social learning theory, and may help to develop self-efficacy in undertaking self-management or caregiver-supported treatment tasks.[30] Feedback from patients/caregiver at one of the author's AD programs[8] strongly indicates that interaction with other patients and caregivers is a valuable and practical experience.

The patient or caregiver needs to show an appropriate level of understanding of when treatment is changed to help ensure good outcomes, such as what action to take if AD becomes infected. An example of a common patient misunderstanding involves the potency and risks versus benefits of topical medications such as topical corticosteroids[32] or topical calcineurin inhibitors.[33–35] It is disappointing that, although we have recognized patient and caregiver phobias and the need for education with respect to underuse of important topical medications, underuse of these agents continues to be one of the key reasons for poor treatment adherence and, in turn, poor therapeutic response. Patients do not understand the pharmaceutical industry's naming and labeling of products. The patient's or caregiver's perception may be that the potency of a corticosteroid or calcineurin inhibitor is based solely on the assigned percent value (ie, 0.05% vs 2.5%), rather than on the specific corticosteroid preparation (ie, beclomethasone dipropionate vs hydrocortisone). This misunderstanding may result in the application of a high-potency corticosteroid (eg, beclomethasone dipropionate 0.05%) to an area of the body such as the face or axillae, and the use of a lower-potency corticosteroid (eg, hydrocortisone 2.5%) to the trunk or extremities, This can be avoided through careful prescription-writing education, including written instructions as to what, where, and when, and review on follow-up.

Another key component of effective educational intervention is the nature and quality of the educational support material aids that are provided, so due regard needs to be given to the quality of evidence-based resources, such as educational booklets or posters (**Fig. 1**, highlighting the different categories of steroid potency as a clinic educational tool) and the use of multimedia resources, such as DVDs or, as highlighted earlier, other technologies such as video.[36]

Work has begun in examining the effectiveness of nurse-led evidence-based education in groups on a large scale to parents of children with AD within the Eczema Educational Program led by Jackson's nursing team at the St John's Institute of Dermatology in London and being evaluated by Ersser's group at Bournemouth University in the United Kingdom.[37] Related work has also been piloted and evaluated in providing systematic and evidence-based, nurse-led support for self-management among adult psoriasis patients, based on an assessment of their support needs. This work has involved the development and use of a self-management learning workbook for use at home, group-learning activity, a DVD reinforcing key points and including a guided relaxation approach to reduce undue stress, development of self-management plans, and a follow-up telephone consultation with the nurse to evaluate learning. Self-management planning is addressed in more detail in **Box 2**, which outlines key education and communication points to be considered in AD management.

AD PATIENTS AND FAMILIES NEED MORE EDUCATION

A study conducted by Cork and colleagues[14] has provided further support for the importance of patient education in improving treatment outcomes in patients with

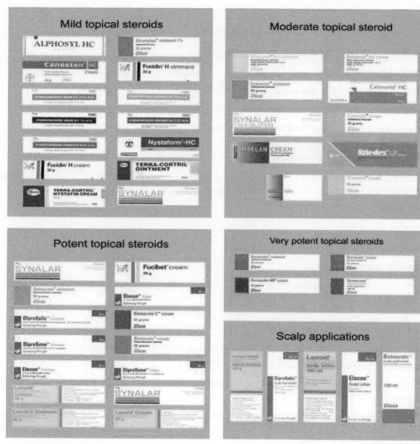

Fig. 1. Topical steroid potencies in the clinic.

AD. Participants included 51 new patients with eczema, ranging in age from 2 weeks to 14 years (mean 4.4 years), who were referred to a dermatologist at a pediatric hospital in Sheffield, England, during a period of approximately 1 year. At baseline, 86% of the patients' parents did not recall ever receiving an explanation of the causes of AD, and 96% had not received any demonstration of how to apply topical treatments. The mean use of emollient cream or ointment at the initial visit was only 54.3 g per week, and 24% of patients were not using any moisturizers. Most (78%) of the patients were using topical corticosteroids, 25% of whom were inappropriately using potent or very potent agents. By the final visit, the patient's mean AD severity score had declined from 42.9 to 4.6. A similar pattern emerged regarding the parents' assessment of eczema severity: the mean score for itching decreased from 7.1 to 1.1, irritability decreased from 5.3 to 0.3, and sleep disturbance decreased from 5.6 to 0.4. The mean weekly use of an emollient cream or ointment increased from 54.3 g to 426 g, whereas the total amount of emollient used increased from 150 g per week to 581 g per week. The increased dose of emollients significantly ($P<.0001$) correlated with the reduction in the AD severity score. During the course of the study, there was increased use of mild corticosteroids and a parallel decline in the use of more potent agents. However, the percentage of patients whose eczema was controlled with emollients alone rose from 0% at visit 1 to 45% at visit 4.

Box 2
Education and communication in AD management

Spend time listening to the patient and/or the parent

Individualize treatment

Explain the nature of the disease and clarify that the goal is control, not cure

Explain the role and the correct use of each therapy, including risks and benefits

Demonstrate the technique and how much of various topical agents to apply (eg, emollients, sealers, medications)

Reinforce the need to use emollients frequently and liberally

Explain the factors that need to be taken into account to decide whether to prescribe topical corticosteroids, topical calcineurin inhibitors, and other systemic therapies:

> Patient's age

> Site to be treated

> Previous response to other therapies

> Extent/severity of disease

Explain how skin infection (bacterial or viral) can cause deterioration in condition, and teach the signs and symptoms of skin infection

Provide written recommendations with step care moving up and down regarding all therapies including bathing and/or showering

Include written instructions for prescription as well as over-the-counter products

Distribute patient-education brochures

Recommend individualized environmental measures to avoid skin irritants and proven allergens

Recommend psychosocial support as appropriate*Adapted from* Nicol NH. Use of moisturizers in dermatologic disease: the role of healthcare providers in optimizing treatment outcomes. Cutis 2005;76(S):30; with permission.

This study and other reviews[15] highlight how patients and caregivers continue to fail to receive adequate information about AD and are not taught properly how to apply topicals, even though instruction and practical demonstrations may be associated with a considerable improvement in treatment outcomes. **Box 2** highlights lessons learned from education and communication in AD management.

AD PATIENT SUPPORT AND RESOURCES

In addition to each provider's AD education tools, it is imperative to offer patients good-quality education resources, otherwise they will find their own, potentially less-reliable resources. Patients with chronic AD may benefit from contacting national patient support organizations. Educational brochures and videos can be obtained from the National Eczema Association in the United States (www.nationaleczema. org) and the National Eczema Society in the United Kingdom (www.eczema.org) (**Box 3**).

Even if the educational information seems to come from reliable sources, it is important to stress to patients and caregivers that they should review advice or tips from outside sources with their treating clinicians. Surridge[38] studied the complex pattern

---

Box 3
International eczema associations: patient support

National Eczema Association (United States)

    4460 Redwood Highway, Suite 16D, San Rafael, CA 94903-1953

    Telephone 415 499 3474 or 800 818 7546

    Web site: www.nationaleczema.org

    E-mail: info@nationaleczema.org

National Eczema Society (United Kingdom)

    Hill House, Highgate Hill, Freepost WC4049, London N19 5NA

    Telephone 020 7281 3553

    Web site: www.eczema.org

    E-mail: info@eczema.org

---

of knowledge sources that parents need to reconcile and the challenges they face when making decisions about their child's eczema management. Even small changes to a treatment regimen can be detrimental or of little benefit, and can add to the cost. An open and ongoing dialog between patients, caregivers, and their clinician improves the likelihood of adherence with the treatment plan and leads to improved outcomes.

ROLE OF NURSES COLLABORATING INTERNATIONALLY TO MOVE AD EDUCATION FORWARD

There is now an urgent need for international collaboration to establish the most effective methods for promoting AD education. Nurses have taken a key role in this area and, as discussed earlier, nurses have made systematic attempts to reveal the evidence gaps in this area and have developed systematic interventions to build effective approaches and the evidence base within this neglected research area. Further efforts should involve international collaboration by nurses and other health professionals, including physicians and clinical psychologists. A key opportunity for nursing collaboration has arisen through the work of the International Skin Care Nursing Group (ISNG; www.isng.org). This article is one example; as co-authors, we are both on the ISNG Advisory Board.

ISNG has sought to develop collaboration among nurses worldwide during the last decade to promote dermatology/skin care nursing, improve educational opportunities for nursing, and encourage development and evaluation. It is affiliated with the International Council of Nurses and is recognized by most of the major international dermatology organizations. ISNG is providing a vehicle for collaboration to achieve a more systematic and evidence-based approach to eczema education and support for using nursing resources. One goal is to highlight the practice development and evaluate the research agenda in this area and the potential for nursing to make a greater contribution in this important field. The international systematic review work, models of good practice such as that for emollient therapy,[28] and appraisal of the existing evidence-based work draws on initiatives and research work by nursing staff; however, there remain many opportunities for multidisciplinary development. In the future, more attention needs to be paid to the cultural relevance of some of these delivery models for application in different regions of the world and to discern which models are congruent with the organization and resources of different health delivery systems.

SUPPORT OF PSYCHOLOGICAL AND EDUCATIONAL INTERVENTIONS

AD affects both adults and children and can be disabling for whole families. Although psychological support and education of the parent/caregiver remain crucial components of disease management, there is inadequate rigorous trial evidence of the effectiveness of educational and psychological interventions when used as an adjunct to topical therapy for childhood AD.[16]

A systematic review of treatments for AD[39] found only limited evidence to support psychological treatments or educational interventions, although a more recent focused review revealed evidence of the value of some planned educational approaches.[16] The latter review examined the effectiveness of educational and psychological interventions in changing outcomes for children with AD. That review was published at the time of NICE[27] guidelines for AD in children[27] and so was not included within it, but it provides a more extensive account of the evidence available, information on the typical service delivery models in use, and an extensive critique of the evidence available (see also the article by Kelsay and colleagues elsewhere in this issue for further exploration of this topic).

The review also examined psychological interventions but found only 1 study that was rigorous enough to meet the inclusion criteria because of the inadequacy of the study designs. Psychological interventions remain virtually unevaluated by studies with robust designs. The only study that was included examined the effect of relaxation techniques, specifically hypnotherapy and biofeedback, on severity.[40] This study found that relaxation techniques improved clinical severity compared with the control at 20 weeks, but this was of borderline significance ($P = .042$).[40]

Psychological interventions are being incorporated into management strategies to reduce scratching behaviors that exacerbate eczema.[41,42] Some of these approaches are behaviorally based, such as behavioral modification. This includes the use of habit reversal in which scratching, an adverse response to the stimulus of pruritus, is replaced by a more adaptive response, such as patting or rubbing the skin. This is preceded by a period of awareness training in which the patient/caregiver keeps a record or diary of the patient's scratching behavior and factors likely to trigger this response.[42–44] For the child with eczema, this may be incorporated into a pattern of play. Nurses are well placed to teach and support patients and caregivers simple behavioral modification techniques and provide psychological support.

In children, the caregiver's ability to manage a child's eczema is an important outcome, and consequently educational or psychological support for parents is required. It could be argued that the general case for psychosocial intervention to improve clinical outcomes in chronic diseases such as AD is well established.[45] However, the evidence in this field of eczema management remains suboptimal, despite some good examples in adult patient support.[46]

In reviewing evidence provided for both psychological and educational support of childhood eczema,[16] one needs to remember that Cochrane systematic reviews by the Cochrane Skin Group only allow the inclusion of findings from randomized controlled trials (RCTs) as the methodology. As such, this may exclude some useful studies, although the evidence base remains limited. All conventional therapies are likely to include a difficult-to-measure level of education that occurs subtly through the care of multiple care providers in addition to any prescribed medications. Most studies were of conventional treatment versus conventional plus psychological/educational, and would be unlikely to find trials examining psychological/educational approaches versus intervention. Furthermore, some interventions that are psychologically or educationally based focus on the parent, the child, or both, and depend on the developmental stage of the child, whereas the outcomes measured often focus on the child and parent. Although some RCTs of therapies have an educational or psychological component, the Cochrane review only included studies in which the educational or psychological intervention was the primary intervention to which the experimental group was exposed.

SUMMARY

Nursing is making a key contribution to the development and evaluation of AD education. Educational interventions have long been recommended and used as a critical adjunct at all levels of therapy for patients with AD to enhance therapy effectiveness. These interventions may be directed toward adult patients or the parent/caregiver or child with eczema, with parents often the primary focus of the educational approaches. Education should be individualized and include teaching about the chronic or relapsing nature of AD, exacerbating factors, and therapeutic options, with benefits, risks, and realistic expectations. This important educational facet of care is becoming increasingly difficult to accomplish and seems to be equally difficult to measure and evaluate. A limited number of studies to date suggest the effectiveness of educational approaches to improve the management of AD, although there are indications of the therapeutic potential of some models of service delivery involving eczema schools and nurse-led approaches on disease severity and quality of life. We recommend that an international priority be given to assessing the effect of patient and parental education by nurses and other care providers in AD management using research studies designed to address the common weaknesses of existing randomized studies. International collaboration will help to establish greater clarity regarding the need for more effective evidence-based models of delivering AD education and support within the health care team.

REFERENCES

1. Kapoor R, Menon C, Hoffstad O, et al. The prevalence of atopic triad in children with physician-confirmed atopic dermatitis. J Am Acad Dermatol 2008;58:68–73.
2. Asher MI, Montefort S, Bjorksten B, et al. Worldwide time trends in the prevalence of symptoms of asthma, allergic rhinoconjunctivitis, and eczema in childhood: ISAAC phase one and three repeat multicountry cross-sectional surveys. Lancet 2006;368:733–43.
3. Boguniewicz M, Abramovits W, Paller A, et al. A multiple-domain framework of clinical, economic, and patient-reported outcomes for evaluating benefits of intervention in atopic dermatitis. J Drugs Dermatol 2007;6:416–23.
4. Herd RM. The morbidity and cost of atopic dermatitis. In: Williams HC, editor. Atopic dermatitis. Cambridge (UK): Cambridge University Press; 2003. p. 85–95.
5. Nicol N, Boguniewicz M. Successful strategies in atopic dermatitis management. Dermatol Nurs 2008;(Suppl):1–19.
6. Boguniewicz M, Nicol N. Conventional therapy for atopic dermatitis. In: Boguniewicz M, editor. Atopic dermatitis. Immunol Allergy Clin North Am 2002;22:107–24
7. Fennessy M, Coupland S, Popay J, et al. The epidemiology and experience of atopic eczema during childhood: a discussion paper on the implications of current knowledge for health care, public health policy and research. J Epidemiol Community Health 2000;54(8):581–9.
8. Boguniewicz M, Nicol N, Kelsay K, et al. A multidisciplinary approach to evaluation and treatment of atopic dermatitis. Semin Cutan Med Surg 2008;27:115–27.
9. Nicol NH. Atopic dermatitis: the (wet) wrap-up. Am J Nurs 1987;87:1560–4.

10. Ben-Gashir MA, Seed PT, Hay RJ, et al. Quality of life and disease severity are correlated in children with atopic dermatitis. Br J Dermatol 2004;150(2): 284–90.
11. Akdis CA, Akdis M, Bieber T, et al. Diagnosis and treatment of atopic dermatitis in children and adults: European Academy of Allergology and Clinical Immunology/ American Academy of Allergy, Asthma and Immunology/PRACTALL consensus report. J Allergy Clin Immunol 2006;118(1):152–69.
12. Bridgett C. Psychodermatology and atopic skin disease in London 1989–1999 – helping patients to help themselves. Dermatol Psychosom 2000;1(4):183–6.
13. Nicol NH, Boguniewicz M. Understanding and treating atopic dermatitis. Nurse Pract Forum 1999;10:48–55.
14. Cork MJ, Britton J, Butler L, et al. Comparison of parent knowledge, therapy utilization and severity of atopic eczema before and after explanation and demonstration of topical therapies by a specialist dermatology nurse. Br J Dermatol 2003;149(3):582–9.
15. Nicol NH. Use of moisturizers in dermatologic disease: the role of healthcare providers in optimizing treatment outcomes. Cutis 2005;76(S):26–31.
16. Ersser SJ, Latter S, Sibley A, et al. Psychological and educational interventions for atopic eczema in children. Cochrane Database Syst Rev 2007;3:CD004054. DOI:10.1002/14651858.CD004054.pub2.
17. Graham-Brown RA, Bourke JF, Bumphrey G. Chinese herbal remedies may contain steroids. BMJ 1994;308(6926):473.
18. Agner T. Compliance among patients with atopic eczema. Acta Derm Venereol Suppl (Stockh) 2005;215:33–5.
19. Staab D, von Rueden U, Kehrt R, et al. Evaluation of a parental training program for the management of childhood atopic dermatitis. Pediatr Allergy Immunol 2002;13(2):84–90.
20. Staab D, Diepgen TL, Fartasch M, et al. Age related, structured educational programmes for the management of atopic dermatitis in children and adolescents: multicentre, randomised controlled trial. BMJ 2006;332(7547):933–8.
21. Niebel G, Kallweit C, Lange I, et al. Direkte versus videovermittelte Elternschulung bei atopischem Ekzem im Kindesalter als Erganzung facharztlicher Behandlung. [Direct versus video-based parental education in the treatment of atopic eczema in children. A controlled pilot study]. Eine Kontrollierte Pilotstudie Hautarzt 2000;51(6):401–11 [in German].
22. Chinn DJ, Poyner T, Sibley G. Randomized controlled trial of a single dermatology nurse consultation in primary care on the quality of life of children with atopic eczema. Br J Dermatol 2002;146(3):432–9.
23. Gradwell C, Thomas KS, English JS, et al. A randomized controlled trial of nurse follow-up clinics: do they help patients and do they free up consultants' time? Br J Dermatol 2002;147:513–7.
24. Brooks J, Ersser SJ, Lloyd A, et al. Nurse-led education sets out to improve patient concordance and prevent recurrence of leg ulcers. J Wound Care 2004;13(3):111–6.
25. National Asthma Education and Prevention Program. Expert panel report 3 (EPR-3): guidelines for the diagnosis and management of asthma-summary report. J Allergy Clin Immunol 2007;120(Suppl 5):S94–138.
26. Ntuen E, Taylor SL, Kinney M, et al. Physicians' perceptions of an eczema action plan for atopic dermatitis. J Dermatolog Treat 2010;21(1):28–33.
27. National Institute for Health and Clinical Excellence. Atopic eczema in children: management of atopic eczema in children from birth up to the age of 12 years.

Available at: http://www.ncc-wch.org.uk/index.asp?PageID=359. 2007. Accessed July 7, 2010.

28. Ersser S, Maguire S, Nicol N, et al. Best practice in emollient therapy: a statement for healthcare professionals, Wounds UK, Ltd. Dermatolog Nurs (Suppl) 2009; 8(3):1–22.

29. Boguniewicz M, Nicol N. General management of patients with atopic dermatitis. In: Reitamo S, Luger TA, Steinhoff M, editors. Textbook of atopic dermatitis. Andover (UK): Informa; 2008. p. 147–64.

30. Bandura A. Self-efficacy: the exercise of control. New York: Freeman; 1997.

31. Long CC, Finlay AY. The finger-tip unit - a new practical measure. Clin Exp Dermatol 1991;16(6):444–7.

32. Nicol NH, Baumeister L. Topical corticosteroid therapy: considerations for prescribing and use. Lippincotts Prim Care Pract 1997;1:62–9.

33. Nicol NH, Boguniewicz M, Hanifin JM, et al. Evolution in the treatment of atopic dermatitis: new approaches to managing a chronic skin disease. Dermatol Nurs 2003;15S(4):3–19.

34. Hultsch T, Kapp A, Spergel J. Immunomodulation and safety of topical calcineurin inhibitors for the treatment of atopic dermatitis. Dermatology 2005;211:174–87.

35. National Institute for Health and Clinical Excellence. Tacrolimus and primecrolimus for atopic eczema. London: National Institute for Clinical Excellence (NICE); 2004.

36. Nicol NH. Managing atopic dermatitis in children and adults. Nurse Pract 2000; 25:58–79.

37. Farasat H, Ersser SJ, Jackson K, et al. Evaluating an eczema education programme in a London borough. Poster presentation at the Inaugural meeting of the Dermatology Nursing Institute. Washington, DC, September 25, 2009.

38. Surridge HR. Exploring parental needs and knowledge when caring for a child with eczema. Exchange (Patient Magazine of the National Eczema Society) no 119;2005. p. 32–3.

39. Hoare C, Li Wan Po A, Williams H. Systematic review of treatments for atopic eczema. Health Technol Assess 2000;4(37):1–191.

40. Sokel B, Christie D. A comparison of hypnotherapy and biofeedback in the treatment of childhood atopic eczema. Contemp Hypn 1993;10(3):145–54.

41. Horne DJ, White AE, Vagos GA. A preliminary study of psychological therapy in the management of atopic eczema. Br J Med Psychol 1989;62(Pt 3):241–8.

42. Giannini AV. Habit reversal technique and eczema. J Allergy Clin Immunol 1997; 100(4):580.

43. Noren P. Habit reversal – a turning point in the treatment of atopic dermatitis. Clin Exp Dermatol 1995;20(1):2–5.

44. Bridgett CP, Noren P. Atopic skin disease: a manual for practitioners. Petersfield (UK): Wrightson Biomedical; 1996.

45. Guevara JP, Wolf FM, Grum CM, et al. Effects of interventions for self management of asthma in children and adolescents: systematic review and meta analysis. BMJ 2003;326(7402):1308–9.

46. Ehlers A, Stangier U, Gieler U. Treatment of atopic dermatitis: a comparison of psychological and dermatological approaches to relapse prevention. J Consult Clin Psychol 1995;63(4):624–35.

Addressing Psychosocial Aspects of Atopic Dermatitis

Kimberly Kelsay, MD[a,b,]*, Mary Klinnert, PhD[a,b],
Bruce Bender, PhD[a,b]

KEYWORDS

- Atopic dermatitis • Behavior • Sleep disturbance
- Adherence • Quality of life • Psychology

Atopic dermatitis (AD) is a common disease estimated to affect between 5% and 15% of children and 3% of adults, often with significant psychological consequences. Onset is often during the first year of life, but the disease can occur throughout childhood and early adulthood. The severity can vary from a small irritating patch to the involvement of extensive areas of the body, with intense pruritus. The clinical course varies but can be chronic or chronic relapsing.

AD has been termed "the rash that itches," a description suggestive of the distress that can accompany this common disease. Although distress has long been recognized, the increasing specificity of the tools used to measure components of the distress associated with AD[1–3] and the objective measures of AD severity[4,5] have enabled investigators to refine knowledge regarding the effect of AD. Families of patients with AD report that quality of life is affected by disease severity, lack of sleep, pruritus and scratching, and the burden of caring for the patient. Although many patients with AD and their caregivers cope well with the disease, there is an increased risk for emotional problems in patients and caregivers, and patients are at an increased risk of having difficulties in sustaining attention. AD clearly can burden and stress families, but stress in turn can affect the illness. Coping is influenced by family factors and disease-specific factors.

There have been significant advances in understanding the pathogenesis and course of AD. Many patients with mild disease are likely to experience remission; however, patients with moderate or severe disease may experience a chronic relapsing course. Although current medical science cannot cure AD, treatment can

[a] Division of Pediatric Behavioral Health, National Jewish Health, 1400 Jackson Street, Denver, CO 80206, USA
[b] Department of Psychiatry, University of Colorado, 13001 East 17th Place, Aurora, Denver, CO 80045, USA
* Corresponding author. Division of Pediatric Behavioral Health, National Jewish Medical and Research Center, 1400 Jackson Street, Suite G311, Denver, CO 80206.
E-mail address: Kelsayk@njhealth.org

Immunol Allergy Clin N Am 30 (2010) 385–396
doi:10.1016/j.iac.2010.05.003
0889-8561/10/$ – see front matter © 2010 Elsevier Inc. All rights reserved.
immunology.theclinics.com

lessen the severity and decrease the frequency of exacerbations. The potential for improvement in the control of AD has increased the possibilities for psychosocial intervention from the limited focus on teaching families and patients how to manage the distress of AD to targeted interventions that may lead to significant gains, such as improved sleep, decreased scratching, and increased adherence with effective treatment. Efficient administration of these interventions is best undertaken within the context of a multidisciplinary team.

This review addresses the present state of knowledge regarding the psychosocial effect of AD and the potential interaction between the family's emotional resources, coping and illness. The components of successful multidisciplinary intervention are also reviewed.

EFFECT OF PEDIATRIC AD ON CHILDREN AND CAREGIVERS

Caring for a child with AD has a major effect on families across a variety of domains. Several investigators have queried children with AD, their parents, and their siblings to determine the specific areas of family life that are affected by this disease.[1,6–8] Parents' concerns have ranged from the practical demands of daily care to sleep deprivation for all family members and the financial burden brought on by treatment costs and other special needs. Chamlin and colleagues[9] documented the effects on 4 domains of functioning for parents and children, including physical health (sleep disruption, itching and related scratching), emotional health (fussiness in children, various emotional stresses for parents), physical functioning (activity restrictions, missed work), and social functioning (feelings of isolation, negative reactions from family members). This wide range of AD-related demands and stresses results in major emotional challenges for parents, affecting their own lives and those of their children, with more severe disease having greater effect on multiple aspects of family functioning.[10]

The practical demands for the daily care required by children with AD consume a great deal of time and energy. In a sample of children treated at a tertiary care center for moderate and severe AD, most parents reported spending about 3 hours each day caring for their child's skin.[11] Parents' care includes getting their children to take bath, accept skin care, avoid allergens and irritants, and ensuring that their child refrains from scratching.[1,6] The difficulties posed by the itching and related scratching are typically the first to be mentioned by parents when they are asked about the effects of their child's AD on their quality of life,[1,6] and managing scratching is the primary concern for parents requesting a pediatric psychology consult.[12] Ratings of itch intensity or pruritus, whether made by parents for young children or by older children for themselves, were significantly and inversely correlated with parents' quality of life, that is, more intense pruritus was related to lower scores for parents' psychosomatic well being, social life, emotional coping, and acceptance of the disease. Older children's self-report of itch intensity was also negatively correlated with their self-report on quality of life and positively correlated with their depressed mood and catastrophic thinking.[13] In addition, higher ratings of child itchiness were related to poorer parent coping with AD, with more aggression related to child scratching, protective behavior, control of scratching, and negative treatment experience.[13] These responses are consistent, with itching skin being the focal experience of AD and the management of itching being the primary coping requirement.[1]

Increased itchiness in children during the night is associated with difficulties in sleeping. Because parents are often up trying to comfort their children and prevent scratching, nighttime sleep deprivation and daytime exhaustion for parents is common, severely affecting their quality of life.[1,14] A study conducted in the United Kingdom investigated the risk factors for AD severity and its effect on quality of life for children aged 5 to 10 years.[15] The investigators found that the most severe effect was sleep disruption in the parents and siblings of the child with AD. Moore and colleagues[16] conducted a comparative questionnaire study of children with AD aged up to 16 years and parents of children the same age with asthma. Results showed that for 2 nights prior to completing the questionnaire, mothers were up for an average of 39 minutes per night and fathers were up for 45 minutes per night; in comparison, parents of children with asthma lost no sleep at all. The time for which mothers were up correlated with their child's age and parent-reported severity of the child's AD. Depression for the mothers of children with AD was 2-fold higher than that for the mothers of children with asthma. Follow-up analyses showed that the mothers' depression scores were related to their sleep disruption rather than to the severity of their child's AD.

Although parents report tremendous effects of their child's AD on their quality of life, research has been mixed as to whether parents' overall psychological functioning is affected. In a study of parents of school-aged children with AD, maternal mental distress was not increased, although parents described themselves as anxious and overprotective.[17] In contrast, in a study of parents of young children with AD, attending an inpatient rehabilitation clinic, high rates of psychological distress were observed in the parents.[18] On the mental health scale of the 12-Item Short Form Health Survey (SF-12®), 39% of the mothers scored greater than a standard deviation less than mean normal values and 15% scored more than 2 SDs less than the healthy norms. Psychosocial distress was the highest for mothers of children with the most severe disease.

In addition to being stressed by demands on their time and exhausted by sleep deprivation, parents report a myriad of anxieties and worries about their children's emotional and behavioral functioning and about how children are coping with their AD. Parents worry about their child's absence at school, attention to academic tasks, and disrupted peer relations.[1] Parents are concerned about their children's behavioral and mood changes and the effects of AD on their children's self-esteem. Parents also express concern about how their child's AD is affecting their relationship with their child, as well as their parenting. Among the parents of preschoolers with AD, mothers felt more stressed in relation to their parenting and less efficient in their disciplining of the affected child, and these mothers had less social support than the mothers of unaffected children.[19] In spite of these worries, the mothers did not display negative attitudes toward their children with AD, and there was no difference in their attachment security between children with AD and normal children. Nevertheless, parents' worries about their children's psychological adjustment are an important source of emotional distress for caregivers of children with AD.

Concerns about financial costs associated with having a child with AD have been noted consistently in response to quality-of-life queries.[1,20] Direct financial costs are derived from purchase of medications and emollients and special foods and supplies, as well as costs related to physician and clinic visits.[21] In addition, indirect costs accrue from the need for parents to take days off from work or because a parent elects not to work to care for the child with AD.[19,21] The rankings of the importance of financial burden relative to other concerns vary by study. For example, financial burdens were the least-frequent concern of families from the United States, responding to the Dermatitis Family Impact (DFI) questionnaire in the 1990s,[1] whereas other researchers reported that according to DFI responses, the greatest effect on the family was on the domains assessing treatment costs.[14] Although the financial burden of AD is very high for the society as a whole,[22] the financial effect for individual families likely depends on factors such as their country, their health care system, and family resources.

ADULT AD

Although less prevalent than pediatric AD, adults who are affected by AD also report negative effects on their quality of life. For example, adults with AD report lower physical role, social functioning, and vitality than adults with psoriasis.[23] Adults with AD report feeling frustrated with their disease and embarrassed and angry about their appearance.[24]

THE RELATIONSHIP BETWEEN AD AND PSYCHOLOGICAL DISORDERS

Although clinical observation and research evidence indicate that psychological distress is increased in patients with AD and in parents of children with AD, it is unclear whether the incidence of actual psychological disorders is increased in this group and, if so, what would be the direction of causality. A single causal direction is often assumed in the relationship between psychological distress and AD, in which the disease is presumed to introduce distress into the life of the patients, driving quality of life downward and psychological dysfunction upward. More probable is a 2-way relationship in which the disease and psychological status are interactive.

AD is clearly a difficult disease for patients and families.[23,25–29] However, results from quality-of-life surveys leave other questions unanswered, such as does feeling distressed by one's disease mean that a psychological disorder is present? Attempts to identify an AD personality trait have generally been unsuccessful; however, increased anxious[24,25,30–33] and depressive symptoms[24,33] have been identified in groups of patients with AD. Elevated symptom scores do not invariably translate into a clear behavioral or mood disorder; rather, the signs of distress falling short of psychopathology characterize many patients with AD.[34,35] A questionnaire study on 108 patients with AD, psoriasis, and severe acne found small but significant differences between these patients and controls, leading to the conclusion that most were experiencing minor psychological distress but that rates of depression and anxiety were not increased.[35] A Canadian survey of 480 patients with facial acne, alopecia areata, AD, and psoriasis reported that suicidal ideation rates were higher in patients with psoriasis and acne when compared with general medical patients (5.6%–7.2% vs 2.4%–3.3%) but not significantly elevated in those with AD,[36] suggesting again that in most cases, psychological distress secondary to the skin disease does not result in clinical psychopathology. At the most-severe end of the AD spectrum, clinical depression and anxiety may be increased, although documentation of a severity-mediated relationship between disease and psychological outcome is scant.[25] In one study 45 patients with AD and 34 health controls completed psychological questionnaires. Patients with disease that was rated as mild demonstrated no increase in test scores, reflecting anxious and depressive symptoms. However, patients with moderate and severe disease demonstrated increased psychological symptoms relative to controls.[25] In another study from Japan, suicidal ideation was reported in 0.21% of patients with mild AD, 6% with moderate disease, and 19.6% with severe disease.[37]

The association between psychological distress and AD does not establish a causal relationship. Intuitively, the increased psychological distress brought on the patient by this disease would seem to account for any increase in distress symptoms. However, at the same time, patients with psychological distress from causes other than their skin disease may experience an exacerbation of their AD. Distressed patients may have increased vulnerability of developing AD or experiencing an exacerbation in their skin condition. Stressful events have often been observed to occur before worsening of symptoms of AD.[38–40] In a study, an AD exacerbation followed a stressful day by 24 hours.[39] One theory emerging from studies of AD and stress posits that adrenocortical response to stress in children with AD is attenuated compared with health controls.[41] Laboratory studies from this research group suggest that patients with AD are more susceptible to stress-induced skin eruptions because of the hyporesponsive hypothalamic-pituitary-adrenal axis that blunts the body's natural ability to produce cortisol and suppresses inflammation in response to stress[42,43] or, alternatively, because of increased reactivity in the sympathetic adrenomedullary system.[44] One study found that in addition to stress increasing the severity of AD, young children with AD who experienced stress were at an increased risk of developing asthma.[45]

Another pathway that might explain the relationship between psychological distress and AD exacerbation addresses the role of treatment adherence. In this case, psychological distress may undermine treatment adherence, and hence may lead to poorer disease control. Depression has been repeatedly associated with declining adherence to treatments for chronic illness.[46–50] The presence of depression in adults with asthma was associated with an 11-fold increase in the odds of nonadherence relative to asthmatic patients without depression.[49] Possibly, because adherence declines as depression increases, depression is associated with a poor prognosis in chronic medical conditions,[51] and in asthma, depression has been specifically linked with increased stay in emergency rooms, hospitalizations, and unscheduled office visits.[52–54]

Nonadherence is also a problem in the treatment of AD. A study of 37 patients with AD included adherence monitoring, using an electronic monitor that recorded each time the medication container was opened.[55] During the 8 weeks of treatment, patients used only 37% of the prescribed doses of their topical antiinflammatory medication. In a similar but smaller study, adherence was monitored in 6 patients with AD.[56] Over a period of 4 weeks, electronic monitoring revealed adherence to topical antiinflammatory medications to be averaging approximately to 50% (range 18%–100%), whereas patients reported approximately 80% adherence (range 71%–100%). Although evidence of a relationship between depressive symptoms and nonadherence in patients with AD is not available, it remains plausible that in this population of patients, as in patients with other chronic illnesses, such a relationship exists and helps to explain the relationship between psychological distress and poor disease outcomes. Because these studies involved children, this relationship may be more complex and involve the emotional state of the parent as well. In support of this result, a study that used parent-reported measures of disease management for AD found that parental mental health, family situation, and disease severity all influenced disease management.[18]

In summary, research data to date support the conclusion that AD decreases quality of life and increases psychological distress, although the incidence of psychological disorders in this population is not likely increased except in those with severe disease. The relationship between psychological distress and AD is most probably interactive; although the presence of AD increases the possibility of psychological distress, the presence of psychological distress also likely causes disease exacerbation either through stress-induced physiologic changes or through declining treatment adherence. Further research is needed to help clarify these relationships. Many of the studies addressing the relationship between AD and psychological functioning have been hampered by several methodological shortcomings, including (1) absence of control subjects; (2) inclusion of control subjects not well matched to index subjects on characteristics that can influence psychological functioning, including age and socioeconomic status; (3) reliance on published normative data from questionnaire development studies rather than a matched control group; and (4) failure to acknowledge that paper-and-pencil questionnaires cannot reliably diagnose psychological disorders and that elevated scores in 1 group does not always indicate psychopathology. Increased understanding of the relationship between AD and psychological functioning will emerge from additional studies that successfully overcome these shortcomings.

THE RELATIONSHIP BETWEEN AD AND SLEEP

Patients with AD are clearly at risk for disturbed sleep. Disturbed sleep is frequently reported by parents of children with AD[20] and adult patients, and it has also been shown using objective measures such as polysomnography.[27] Although as a group, patients with AD correctly note that they are sleeping poorly, at least 2 studies have shown that self-reported measures of sleep quality do not correlate with objective measures of sleep for adults with AD.[27,57] Similarly, a study comparing subjective report of sleep difficulty with objective signs of AD severity in children found no correlation.[58] Scratching during sleep has been measured using actigraphy[57,59] and infrared video monitoring[60] and is associated with disturbed sleep, but scratching may not account for the whole of sleep disturbance that is associated with AD.[61] Regardless of the cause, sleep disturbance affects not only the quality of life but also the cognitive function and behavior. In children who do not have AD, poor sleep has been associated with increased behavioral problems at home[62] and at school[63] and poor attention span.[64] The relationship between sleep and attention-deficit/hyperactivity disorder (ADHD) for children with AD was examined in a large population-based study.[65] Children with AD were compared with age-sex–matched controls without AD. Children with AD were at increased risk of being diagnosed with ADHD only if they also had a sleep disturbance.

AD AND COMORBID ATOPIC ILLNESS

Studies that have examined the psychosocial effect of AD have either used populations without comorbid atopic illness or have not described the extent of the comorbid illness in the population studied. A significant number of children with AD may also have asthma and allergies.[66] Approximately 40% of children with AD may have food allergies (see also the article by Caubet and Eigenmann elsewhere in this issue for further exploration of this topic).[67] There is substantial literature regarding the negative effect of asthma and food allergies on quality of life, and comorbid illness may increase the negative effect of AD. However, the potentiated effect of AD on the quality of life, behavioral and emotional health of children, and families in the presence of comorbid atopic illness remains to be sufficiently studied.

INTERVENTION

Treatment of AD is complex, with education being a key component. There is evidence to support brief multidisciplinary education of parents and children with AD[68] as well as longer interventions. In a large multicenter trial for children with AD, over 900 patients, aged 3 months to 18 years, were randomized to either a wait group or a 6 week intervention group with weekly 2 hour education sessions.[69] A pediatrician provided general information about AD, daily skin care, recognition and avoidance of triggers, and unconventional therapies. A nutritionist covered topics on food allergies, nutrition, and diet; a psychologist taught relaxation, coping, self-management, and dealing with itching, scratching, and sleep. Children were divided into 3 groups: younger than 7 years (only parents attended the groups), 8 to 12 years (parents and children attended), and 13 to 18 years (only the youth attended the groups). At 12-months follow-up, children of all ages in the intervention groups showed improvements in AD severity compared with the control group, and parents of children aged 3 months to 7 years showed improvements in quality of life on all dimensions, whereas parents of children aged 8 to 12 years showed improvements in emotional coping and confidence in medical team. Children also showed some improvements in coping with scratching.[69] Another randomized study used a similar intervention in a sample of 204 families of children with AD (aged 5 months–12 years) and found improvements in treatment adherence and treatment costs in the intervention group compared with the control group.[70]

These education sessions were provided on an outpatient basis to children with moderate to severe AD. Another treatment model is to incorporate multidisciplinary care within a day treatment program for children who have failed outpatient care. Opportunities exist to expand treatment targets and expand the model of service delivery within this setting. The multidisciplinary team consists of allergist-immunologists, nurses, child life professionals, creative arts therapists, social workers, pediatric psychologists, and child and adolescent psychiatrists. Within this setting, the improvement is often dramatic,[71] and families often accept and engage in multidisciplinary intervention. The ultimate goal of multidisciplinary care for children with AD is to give the family and the child tools to control symptoms at home and to improve the child's future quality of life. A study of 50 children with AD found that parents reported sustained improvements in both symptoms of AD and quality of life over the course of 2 years after treatment at the authors' center.[72] In this setting, patients receive a comprehensive evaluation, treatment, and education over 5 to 10 days. Caregivers are taught skin care and hydration therapy (baths and wet wraps) within the context of treatment; they initially observe the nurse provide care and then perform the care themselves with the guided supervision of experienced nursing staff (see the article by Nicol and Ersser elsewhere in this issue for further exploration of this issue).

Child life professionals and creative arts therapists use developmentally appropriate tools to help the child cope with procedures and minimize psychological trauma. The child life specialists help the child through the first few baths, which can be uncomfortable and anxiety provoking, by using techniques such as gently engaging and distracting the child. Each child is given their own set of bath toys to take home, and child life professionals model for parents in how to engage children in distracting activities while remaining calm. The creative arts specialist runs a daily group focused on acclimatizing children to their treatment and helping them understand their feelings about themselves and their illness. Techniques include giving the child a doll, which they are told shares their likes, dislikes, and illness.[71] The child decorates the doll and marks the regions of the skin affected by AD. The child is asked to help the doll feel safe and help the doll's skin get better. The child gives the doll a symbolic bath, applies ointments, and wraps the affected regions. Children often act more protectively and caringly toward their doll than they have been able to toward themselves. Parents attend a daily discussion session led by either a social worker or a psychologist. The topics include interacting with systems such as the schools and medical systems, managing outside activities, siblings, parenting, sleep, and breaking the itch-scratch cycle. Parents benefit from interacting with other parents who share some of their challenges.

Each patient (and family unit) is assigned a psychosocial clinician (social worker or pediatric psychologist) on arrival, who performs a behavioral health assessment of the family's and child's coping and response to illness. Treatment is then tailored to the needs of the family and varies from supportive psychoeducational care to more intensive daily therapy focused on marital issues, anger, guilt, and so forth. Minimizing scratching is a treatment goal that the child is able to engage in more readily because their AD typically improves within 48 to 72 hours. Techniques include distraction, replacement, biofeedback, and hypnosis, depending on the age and psychology of the child. The psychosocial clinician communicates any recommendations for further action or mental health care to the family and referring physician within a written home-care plan and any recommendations for school accommodations to the family and the school within a written school care plan.[71]

The psychiatrist is available for consultations. Questions typically concern sleep, diagnostic considerations and treatment options for anxiety, irritability, poor focus, and depression. Medications to help with sleep are often needed for the first few days but can often be rapidly tapered as the skin improves.[73] As sleep, skin inflammation, and scratching improve, the child often demonstrates a dramatic change in affect. For this reason consultations regarding mood and behavior are often held until later in the admission. Another consultation question concerns sedation for the first baths, which can be very uncomfortable and anxiety provoking. The authors recommend avoiding sedation, given proper nursing and psychosocial support for baths, because children rapidly acclimatize without sedation and the authors do not want to inadvertently communicate to the family and child that they will not be able to manage severe AD exacerbations at home.

The medical and psychosocial teams meet weekly to discuss each patient, their response to treatment, plan further care, and strategize regarding any problems. This meeting helps to ensure that families receive a consistent message from the

---

Box 1
Key points regarding psychosocial care

1. Moderate to severe AD negatively affects patients and their families.

2. Pruritus, scratching, and sleep problems are common complaints linked to impaired quality of life.

3. Treatment is complex and nonadherence rates are high.

4. Multidisciplinary interventions have shown success in improving treatment adherence, quality of life, and disease severity.

5. Families and patients should demonstrate skin care techniques because this often reveals problems in their understanding of AD management.

6. Managing distress around procedures is an important element of treatment that can usually be achieved without sedation.

7. Within a treatment setting, assessing psychopathology such as depression, anxiety, and ADHD is best undertaken after treatment of AD begins and acute inflammation is decreased.

8. Children can engage in managing scratching when they are not suffering from an acute exacerbation, but during an exacerbation, treatment should first focus on improving AD.

9. Sleep medication may be needed during an exacerbation.

10. Written home care plans for treatment of varying levels of severity of AD are helpful for families, and for the child who attends school, a school care plan should be included.

entire team and prevents miscommunication and more serious problems such as splitting. The team also meets with the family to review progress and address any issues. At discharge key members from the team attend a formal meeting with the family to present and discuss the written home care plan and address final questions.

SUMMARY

AD, especially moderate to severe, can have significant negative effect on patients and their families. Although this illness does not typically cause psychological disorders, it is highly distressing for children, parents, and adults. Successful treatment includes assessing and treating AD and engaging families in the complex care needed to manage illness. Evidence supports multidisciplinary intervention aimed at empowering families because they take on the many tasks associated with chronic illness. Successful teams are able to ally with patients and families to build a realistic shared optimism for the future (**Box 1**).

REFERENCES

1. Lawson V, Lewis-Jones M, Finlay A, et al. The family of childhood atopic dermatitis: the Dermatitis Family Impact Questionnaire. Br J Dermatol 1998;138:107–13.
2. Reid P, Lewis-Jones MS. Sleep difficulties and their management in preschoolers with atopic eczema. Clin Exp Dermatol 1995;20:38–41.
3. Finlay A, Khan G. Dermatology Life Quality Index (DLQI)–a simple practical measure for routine clinical use. Clin Exp Dermatol 1994;19:210–6.
4. Carel K, Bratton DL, Miyazawa N, et al. The Atopic Dermatitis Quickscore (ADQ): validation of a new parent-administered atopic dermatitis scoring tool. Ann Allergy Asthma Immunol 2008;101:500–7.
5. Severity scoring of atopic dermatitis: the SCORAD index. Consensus report of the European Task Force on Atopic Dermatitis. Dermatology 1993;186:23–31.
6. Chamlin SL, Frieden IJ, Williams ML, et al. Effects of atopic dermatitis on young American children and their families. Pediatrics 2004;114:607–11.
7. McKenna S, Whalley D, Dewar A, et al. International development of the Parents' Index of Quality of Life in Atopic Dermatitis (PIQoL-AD). Qual Life Res 2005;14:231–41.
8. Von Ruden U, Kehrt R, Stabb D, et al. Development and validation of a disease specific questionnaire on quality of life of parents of children with atopic dermatitis. Z Gesundheitswiss 1999;4:335–50.
9. Chamlin SL, Cella D, Frieden IJ, et al. Development of the Childhood Atopic Dermatitis Impact Scale: initial validation of a quality-of-life measure for young children with atopic dermatitis and their families. J Invest Dermatol 2005;125:1106–11.
10. Balkrishnan R, Housman T, Carroll C, et al. Disease severity and associated family impact in childhood atopic dermatitis. Arch Dis Child 2003;88:423–7.
11. Kaugars AS, Klinnert MD, Price MR, et al. Physical and psychosocial functioning of children with atopic dermatitis. J Allergy Clin Immunol 2003;111:A347.
12. LeBovidge JS, Kelley SD, Lauretti A, et al. Integrating medical and psychological health care for children with atopic dermatitis. J Pediatr Psychol 2007;32:617–25.
13. Weisshaar E, Diepgen TL, Bruckner T, et al. Itch intensity evaluated in the German Atopic Dermatitis Intervention Study (GADIS): correlations with quality of life, coping behaviour and SCORAD severity in 823 children. Acta Derm Venereol 2008;88:234–9.

14. Alvarenga T, Caldeira A. Quality of life in pediatric patients with atopic dermatitis. J Pediatr (Rio J) 2009;85:415–20.
15. Ben-Gashir M, Seed P, Hay R. Are quality of family life and disease severity related in childhood atopic dermatitis? J Eur Acad Dermatol Venereol 2002;16: 455–62.
16. Moore K, David T, Murray C, et al. Effect of childhood eczema and asthma on parental sleep and well-being: a prospective comparative study. Br J Dermatol 2006;154:514–8.
17. Absolon C, Cottrell D, Eldridge SM, et al. Psychological disturbance in atopic eczema: the extent of the problem in school-aged children. Br J Dermatol 1997;137:241–5.
18. Warschburger P, Buchholz HT, Petermann F. Psychological adjustment in parents of young children with atopic dermatitis: which factors predict parental quality of life? Br J Dermatol 2004;150:304–11.
19. Daud L, Garralda M, David T. Psychosocial adjustment in preschool children with atopic eczema. Arch Dis Child 1993;69:670–6.
20. Chamlin SL, Mattson CL, Frieden IJ, et al. The price of pruritus: sleep disturbance and cosleeping in atopic dermatitis. Arch Pediatr Adolesc Med 2005; 159:745–50.
21. Su JC, Kemp AS, Varigos GA, et al. Atopic eczema: its impact on the family and financial cost. Arch Dis Child 1997;76:159–62.
22. Mancini A, Kaulback K, St M, et al. The socioeconomic impact of atopic dermatitis in the United States: a systematic review. Pediatr Dermatol 2008;25:1–6.
23. Kiebert G, Sorensen SV, Revicki D, et al. Atopic dermatitis is associated with a decrement in health-related quality of life. Int J Dermatol 2002;41:151–8.
24. Linnet J, Jemec GB. An assessment of anxiety and dermatology life quality in patients with atopic dermatitis. Br J Dermatol 1999;140:268–72.
25. Hashiro M, Okumura J. Anxiety, depression and psychosomatic symptoms in patients with atopic dermatitis: comparison with normal controls and among groups of different degrees of severity. J Dermatol Sci 1997;14:63–7.
26. Zachariae R, Zachariae C, Ibsen H, et al. Psychological symptoms and quality of life of dermatology outpatients and hospitalized dermatology patients. Acta Derm Venereol 2004;84:205–12.
27. Bender B, Ballard R, Canono B, et al. Disease severity, scratching, and sleep quality in patients with atopic dermatitis. J Am Acad Dermatol 2008;58:415–20.
28. Hon K, Leung T, Wong K, et al. Does age or gender influence quality of life in children with atopic dermatitis? Clin Exp Dermatol 2008;33:705.
29. Brenninkmeijer E, Legierse C, Sillevis Smitt J, et al. The course of life of patients with childhood atopic dermatitis. Pediatr Dermatol 2009;26:14–22.
30. Buske-Kirschbaum A, Ebrecht M, Kern S, et al. Personality characteristics in chronic and non-chronic allergic conditions. Brain Behav Immun 2008;22:762–8.
31. Garrie S, Garrie E. Anxiety and skin diseases. Cutis 1978;22:205–8.
32. Habib S, Morrissey S. Stress management for atopic dermatitis. Behav Change 1999;16:226–36.
33. Shirata K, Nishitani Y, Kawahira K. Study on the mental health of patients with atopic dermatitis in adults. Osaka City Med J 1995;41:75–83.
34. Misery L, Thomas L, Jullien D, et al. Comparative study of stress and quality of life in outpatients consulting for different dermatoses in 5 academic departments of dermatology. Eur J Dermatol 2008;18:412–5.
35. Magin P, Pond C, Smith W, et al. A cross-sectional study of psychological morbidity in patients with acne, psoriasis and atopic dermatitis in specialist

dermatology and general practices. J Eur Acad Dermatol Venereol 2008;22: 1435–44.

36. Gupta M, Gupta A. Depression and suicidal ideation in dermatology patients with acne, alopecia areata, atopic dermatitis and psoriasis. Br J Dermatol 1998;139: 846–50.

37. Kimata H. Prevalence of suicidal ideation in patients with atopic dermatitis. Suicide Life Threat Behav 2006;36:120–4.

38. Brown D. Stress as a precipitant factor of eczema. J Psychosom Res 1972;16: 321–7.

39. King R, Wilson G. Use of diary technique to investigate psychosomatic relations in atopic dermatitis. J Psychosom Res 1991;35:697–706.

40. Lammintautsta K, Kalimo K, Raitala R. Prognosis of atopic dermatitis: a prospective study in early adulthood. Int J Dermatol 1991;30:563–8.

41. Buske-Kirschbaum A, Jobst S, Psych D, et al. Attenuated free cortisol response to psychosocial stress in children with atopic dermatitis. Psychosom Med 1997; 59:419–26.

42. Buske-Kirschbaum A, Geiben A, Hollig H, et al. Altered responsiveness of the hypothalamus-pituitary-adrenal axis and the sympathetic adrenomedullary system to stress in patients with atopic dermatitis. Acta Paediatr 2002;87:4245–51.

43. Buske-Kirschbaum A, von Auer K, Krieger S, et al. Blunted cortisol responses to psychosocial stress in asthmatic children: a general feature of atopic disease? Psychosom Med 2003;65:806–10.

44. Buske-Kirschbaum A, Ebrecht M, Kern S, et al. Endocrine stress responses in TH1-mediated chronic inflammatory skin disease (psoriasis vulgaris)—do they parallel stress-induced endocrine changes in TH2-mediated inflammatory dermatoses (atopic dermatitis)? Psychoneuroendocrinology 2006;31: 439–46.

45. Stevenson J. Relationship between behavior and asthma in children with atopic dermatitis. Psychosom Med 2003;65:971–5.

46. McKellar J, Humphreys K, Piette J. Depression increases diabetes symptoms by complicating patients' self-care adherence. Diabetes Educ 2004;30:485–92.

47. Put C, Van den Bergh O, Demedts M, et al. A study of the relationship among self-reported noncompliance, symptomatology, and psychological variables in patients with asthma. J Asthma 2000;37:503–10.

48. Dimatteo R, Lepper H, Croghan T. Depression is a risk factor for noncompliance with medical treatment: meta-analysis of the effects of anxiety and depression on patient adherence. Arch Intern Med 2000;160:2101–7.

49. Smith A, Krishnan J, Bilderback A, et al. Depressive symptoms and adherence to asthma therapy after hospital discharge. Chest 2006;130:1034–8.

50. Bartlett S, Krishnan J, Riekert K. Maternal depressive symptoms and adherence to therapy in inner-city children with asthma. Pediatrics 2004;113:229–37.

51. Katon W. Clinical and health services relationships between major depression, depressive symptoms and general medical illness. Biol Psychiatry 2003;54: 216–26.

52. Mancuso C, Rincon M, McCulloch C, et al. Self-efficacy, depressive symptoms, and patients' expectations predict outcomes in asthma. Med Care 2001;39:1326–38.

53. Eisner M, Katz P, Lactao G, et al. Impact of depressive symptoms on adult asthma outcomes. Ann Allergy Asthma Immunol 2005;94:566–74.

54. Richardson L, Russo J, Lozano P, et al. The effect of comorbid anxiety and depressive disorders on health care utilization and costs among adolescents with asthma. Gen Hosp Psychiatry 2008;30:398–406.

55. Krejci-Manwaring J, Tusa M, Carroll C, et al. Stealth monitoring of adherence to topical medication: adherence is very poor in children with atopic dermatitis. J Am Acad Dermatol 2007;56:1–9.

56. Conde J, Kaur M, Fleischer AJ, et al. Adherence to clocortolone pivalate cream 0.1% in a pediatric population with atopic dermatitis. Cutis 2008;81:435–41.

57. Bringhurst C, Waterston K, Schofield O, et al. Measurement of itch using actigraphy in pediatric and adult populations. J Am Acad Dermatol 2004;51:893–8.

58. Hon KL, Leung TF, Wong Y, et al. Lesson from performing SCORADs in children with atopic dermatitis: subjective symptoms do not correlate well with disease extent or intensity. Int J Dermatol 2006;45:728–30.

59. Bender BG, Leung SB, Leung DY. Actigraphy assessment of sleep disturbance in patients with atopic dermatitis: an objective life quality measure. J Allergy Clin Immunol 2003;111:598–602.

60. Ebata T, Aizawa H, Kamide R. An infrared video camera system to observe nocturnal scratching in atopic dermatitis patients. J Dermatol 1996;23:153–5.

61. Reuveni H, Chapnick G, Tal A, et al. Sleep fragmentation in children with atopic dermatitis. Arch Pediatr Adolesc Med 1999;153:249–53.

62. Lavigne JV, Arend R, Rosenbaum D, et al. Sleep and behavior problems among preschoolers. J Dev Behav Pediatr 1999;20:164–9.

63. Bates JE, Viken RJ, Alexander DB, et al. Sleep and adjustment in preschool children: sleep diary reports by mothers relate to behavior reports by teachers. Child Dev 2002;73:62–74.

64. Chervin RD, Ruzicka DL, Giordani BJ, et al. Sleep-disordered breathing, behavior, and cognition in children before and after adenotonsillectomy. Pediatrics 2006;117:e769–778.

65. Romanos M, Gerlach M, Warnke A, et al. Association of attention-deficit/hyperactivity disorder and atopic eczema modified by sleep disturbance in a large population-based sample. J Epidemiol Community Health 2010;64:269–73.

66. Kjaer HF, Eller E, Host A, et al. The prevalence of allergic diseases in an unselected group of 6-year-old children. The DARC birth cohort study. Pediatr Allergy Immunol 2008;19:737–45.

67. Hauk PJ. The role of food allergy in atopic dermatitis. Curr Allergy Asthma Rep 2008;8:188–94.

68. Grillo M, Gassner L, Marshman G, et al. Pediatric atopic eczema: the impact of an educational intervention. Pediatr Dermatol 2006;23:428–36.

69. Staab D, Diepgen TL, Fartasch M, et al. Age related, structured educational programmes for the management of atopic dermatitis in children and adolescents: multicentre, randomised controlled trial. BMJ 2006;332:933–8.

70. Staab D, von Rueden U, Kehrt R, et al. Evaluation of a parental training program for the management of childhood atopic dermatitis. Pediatr Allergy Immunol 2002;13:84–90.

71. Boguniewicz M, Nicol N, Kelsay K, et al. A multidisciplinary approach to evaluation and treatment of atopic dermatitis. Semin Cutan Med Surg 2008;27:115–27.

72. Kelsay K, Carel D, Bratton DL, et al. Functional status following treatment of children with atopic dermatitis. J Allergy Clin Immunol 2006;117:s233.

73. Kelsay K. Management of sleep disturbance associated with atopic dermatitis. J Allergy Clin Immunol 2006;118:198–201.

Vitamin D in Atopic Dermatitis, Asthma and Allergic Diseases

Daniel A. Searing, MD[a], Donald Y.M. Leung, MD, PhD[b,c],*

KEYWORDS

• Vitamin D • Atopic dermatitis • Asthma • Allergy

Observations by Sniadecki and Palm of the lower prevalence of rickets in rural and equatorial populations, respectively, prompted both investigators to hypothesize that sun exposure was the reason for such a difference.[1–3] Subsequent work by Mellanby[4] established cod liver oil as a cure for dogs with rickets and experiments by McCollum and colleagues[5] demonstrated the existence of a vitamin within cod liver oil. Cod liver oil and sunlight exposure became known as treatment modalities for rickets. Foods containing cholesterol that were irradiated with light were also shown to cure rickets. Windaus and colleagues[6] subsequently discovered a cholesterol precursor, 7-dehydrocholesterol (7-DHC). Their Nobel Prize winning work showed that irradiation of 7-DHC with UV light induced formation of vitamin D_3.[1]

Humans receive at least 80% of their vitamin D through UV-induced skin production.[7,8] According to the Environmental Protection Agency's National Human Activity Pattern Survey (NHAPS), 95% of Americans work indoors.[9] In addition, Americans spend only 10% of available daylight hours outside. One recent study found that during their time outdoors, Americans are exposed to 30% of the available ambient UV light secondary to conditions such as shade.[9] A similar study again using NHAPS data found that children and adolescents spend the same amount of time outside as adults (10% of the day). However, adolescents receive the lowest UV dose of any group.[10] Furthermore, the use of sunscreen with a sun protection factor of 8 decreases cutaneous vitamin D production by 97.5%.[7]

This work is supported by NIH Grants AR 41256 and N01 AI 40029.

[a] Division of Pediatric Allergy and Immunology, Department of Pediatrics, National Jewish Health, 1400 Jackson Street, K731a, Denver, CO 80206, USA

[b] Division of Pediatric Allergy and Immunology, National Jewish Health, 1400 Jackson Street, K926i, Denver, CO 80206, USA

[c] Department of Pediatrics, University of Colorado Denver, The Children's Hospital, 13123 East 16th Avenue, B065, Aurora, CO 80045, USA

* Corresponding author. Division of Pediatric Allergy and Immunology, National Jewish Health, 1400 Jackson Street, K926i, Denver, CO 80206.

E-mail address: leungd@njhealth.org

Immunol Allergy Clin N Am 30 (2010) 397–409

doi:10.1016/j.iac.2010.05.005

0889-8561/10/$ – see front matter © 2010 Elsevier Inc. All rights reserved.

immunology.theclinics.com

Data from the National Health and Nutrition Examination Survey (NHANES) from 2001 to 2004 have shown that, overall, sufficient levels of vitamin D were present in less than a quarter of the adolescent and adult US population studied.[11] More recently, NHANES data looking at children found that 61% of subjects aged 1 to 21 years were vitamin D insufficient.[12] However, there are potential issues with the validity of the assay used for vitamin D data from NHANES. According to the Center for Disease Control and Prevention Web site, 25-hydroxyvitamin D (the main indicator of the body's vitamin D status as discussed later) data from the 2000 to 2006 NHANES was likely affected by drifts in the assay performance over time.[13] In a group of patients ages 0 to 18 years with asthma, atopic dermatitis, and/or food allergy, our group has noted 48% of patients with insufficient (<30 ng/mL) levels of serum 25-hydroxyvitamin D (also referred to as 25(OH)D in the literature and referred to as just vitamin D hereafter unless being discussed in the context of metabolism).[14]

Data in adults suggest that vitamin D levels less than approximately 30 ng/mL are associated with changes in parathyroid hormone levels, as well as intestinal calcium transport.[8] This has led some to argue that vitamin D levels between 20 and 30 ng/mL be considered vitamin D insufficient, although no consensus on optimal vitamin D levels exists.[8] A recent clinical report from the American Academy of Pediatrics changed the recommended dosage of vitamin D from 200 to 400 IU per day for all children (infants to adolescents).[15] Typically, infant and child multivitamin and vitamin D preparations contain 400 IU per dose of vitamin D in either D_2 or D_3 form (see later discussion). The report cites information from adult studies that have helped create the concept of serum vitamin D insufficiency. The Food and Nutrition Board has convened an expert committee to revisit the dietary reference intake for vitamin D and its report is expected to be released in May 2010.[16] Despite these new recommendations, there is concern that intake of 400 IU per day of vitamin D remains inadequate to promote sufficient levels of vitamin D and that the tolerable upper intake level of vitamin D can safely be increased.[17] Graded oral dosing of adults showed that an 8-week course of 400 IU per day of vitamin D_3 raises the serum vitamin D concentration by only 4.4 ng/mL.[18]

Although the relationship between vitamin D deficiency and rickets is well established, only more recently has the role of vitamin D deficiency and insufficiency in allergic disease been debated. Before allergic disease entered the debate, epidemiologic research described links between vitamin D and cancer, type 1 diabetes, and multiple sclerosis.[8,19] The International Study of Asthma and Allergies in Childhood (ISAAC) found the highest prevalence of asthma symptoms in countries such as the United Kingdom, Australia, New Zealand, and the Republic of Ireland.[20] These data helped form the foundation for the description that people living in more westernized, developed nations have higher reported rates of asthma, atopic dermatitis, and hay fever.[21] Studies in various Chinese cities with different socioeconomic profiles found the greatest amount of asthma and allergic symptoms in Hong Kong, the most westernized city studied.[22] Different investigators have hypothesized that westernization, a lifestyle likely to be associated with greater time spent indoors, has fostered a propensity for vitamin D deficiency, which in turn has resulted in more asthma and allergy.[19,23] The scientific evidence for this hypothesis is reviewed.

VITAMIN D METABOLISM

Vitamin D enters the body through either the skin via cutaneous conversion of 7-DHC into pre-vitamin D_3 or the gut via food and/or supplement ingestion (**Fig. 1**).[8] 7-DHC is converted into pre-vitamin D_3 by solar UV B radiation.[8] Sunlight also converts

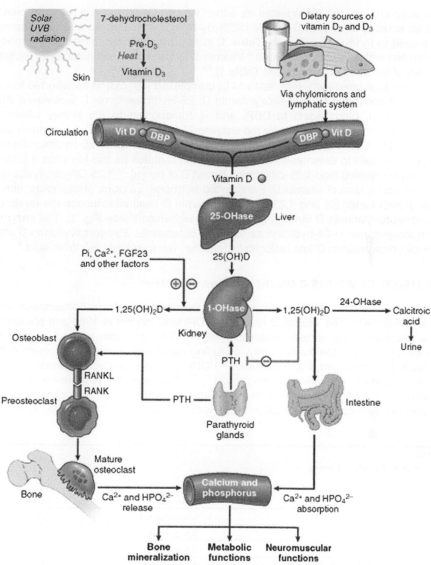

Fig. 1. Vitamin D metabolism. Vitamin D is produced from 7-dehydrocholesterol in the skin or is ingested in the diet. It is converted in the liver into 25-hydroxyvitamin D, and in kidney into 1,25-dihydroxyvitamin D, the active form of the vitamin. 1,25-Dihydroxyvitamin D stimulates the expression of RANKL, an important regulator of osteoclast maturation and function, on osteoblasts, and enhances the intestinal absorption of calcium and phosphorus in the intestine. DBP, vitamin D–binding protein (α1-globulin). (*From* Kumar V, Abbas AK, Fausto N, et al. Environmental and nutritional diseases. In: Robbins and Cotran pathologic basis of disease. 8th edition. Philadelphia: Saunders/Elsevier; 2010. p. 434; with permission.)

pre-vitamin D_3 and/or vitamin D_3 into inert products to prevent vitamin D intoxication.[8] Pre-vitamin D_3 isomerizes to vitamin D_3, is transferred to the dermal capillaries, and binds with vitamin D–binding protein (DBP).[24] Ingested vitamin D uses chylomicrons and the lymphatic system for transportation to the circulation (see **Fig. 1**). Vitamin D from supplements can be ingested as either vitamin D_2 (ergocalciferol) from plant-derived sources or vitamin D_3 (cholecalciferol) from animal-derived sources. Vitamin D_3 is used to fortify several foods (**Table 1**) in the United States, although few foods are fortified with vitamin D in Europe.[8] Vitamin D is also contained naturally in several species of fish and cod liver oil (see **Table 1**).[24]

Vitamin D_3 (subsequently referred to as D) complexed with DBP is transported to the liver and is converted to 25-hydroxyvitamin D. 25-Hydroxyvitamin D is released into the circulation, binds again to DBP, and is transported to the kidney where it undergoes further hydroxylation by the enzyme 25-hydroxyvitamin D-1 α-hydroxylase (CYP27B1) to 1,25-dihydroxyvitamin D or 1,25$(OH)_2$D (see **Fig. 1**). 25-Hydroxyvitamin D levels are used to determine the body's vitamin D status as this form has a longer half-life (2–3 weeks) than 1,25-dihydroxyvitamin D (4 hours).[24] 1,25-Dihydroxyvitamin D is the active form of vitamin D. Parathyroid hormone, calcium, phosphorus, fibroblast growth factor 23, and 1,25-dihydroxyvitamin D itself all influence the levels of 1,25-dihydroxyvitamin D through a variety of mechanisms (see **Fig. 1**). The enzyme 25-hydroxyvitamin D-24-hydroxylase (CYP24) catabolizes 25-hydroxyvitamin D and 1,25-dihydroxyvitamin D into biologically inactive, water-soluble calcitroic acid.[8]

THE EFFECTS OF VITAMIN D ON THE IMMUNE SYSTEM

The scope of vitamin D's biologic actions go beyond just calcium homeostasis and bone metabolism. The vitamin D receptor (VDR) was cloned in 1988 and shown to be a member of the nuclear receptor family.[25] VDR has been located in multiple tissues and cells in the human body, including peripheral blood mononuclear cells (PBMCs) and activated T lymphocytes.[26] VDRs are also located on dendritic cells (DCs), important antigen-presenting cells.[27,28] The enzyme responsible for the synthesis of 1,25-dihydroxyvitamin D, 25-hydroxyvitamin D-1-α-hydroxylase, is located on macrophages and DCs.[29] 25-Hydroxyvitamin D-24-hydroxylase, which

Table 1
Vitamin D content of foods

Food	Amount	Vitamin D Content (IU)
Cod liver oil	1 tablespoon	1360
Salmon, cooked	3.5 ounces	360
Mackerel, cooked	3.5 ounces	345
Sardines, canned in oil, drained	1.75 ounces	250
Tuna fish, canned in oil	3 ounces	200
Milk, vitamin D-fortified	1 cup	98
Margarine, fortified	1 tablespoon	60
Ready-to-eat cereal, fortified with 10% of the daily value for vitamin D	0.75–1 cup	40
Egg, whole	1	20
Liver, beef	3.5 ounces	15
Cheese, Swiss	1 ounce	12

Adapted from http://dietary-supplements.info.nih.gov/factsheets/vitamind.asp#h3. Office of Dietary Supplements, National Institutes of Health. U.S. Department of Agriculture, Agricultural Research Service. USDA Nutrient Database for Standard Reference, Release 21, 2009, Table 3.

degrades 1,25-dihydroxyvitamin D, is also found in monocytes and macrophages.[30] Normal T and B lymphocytes have been shown to express the vitamin D receptor after activation with phytohemagglutinin and Ebstein-Barr virus.[31]

Further research has shown that vitamin D has multiple cytokine-modulating effects through several different cells of the immune system. Tsoukas and colleagues[32] showed that picomolar concentrations of 1,25-dihydroxyvitamin D decreased IL-2 activity and inhibited the proliferation of mitogen-activated lymphocytes. Mahon and colleagues[33] showed that quiescent CD4$^+$ T cells, in addition to activated T cells, expressed VDRs. Furthermore, 1,25-dihydroxyvitamin D decreased proliferation of Th1 and Th2 cells, and lowered the production of interferon (IFN)-γ, interleukin (IL)-2, and IL-5. In contrast, IL-4 production by Th2 cells was increased by 1,25-dihydroxyvitamin D.[33] Froicu and colleagues[34] performed experiments with VDR knockout (KO) mice. Compared with wild-type (WT) mice, VDR KO mice produced more IFN-γ. However, VDR KO mice also produced less IL-2, IL-4, and IL-5 than WT mice. Boonstra and colleagues[35] showed that vitamin D inhibits IFN-γ production and promotes IL-4, IL-5, and IL-10 production in a mouse model. These studies suggest that deficiencies in vitamin D levels and/or signaling would favor a predominant Th1 response and that the presence of vitamin D, although suppressing Th1 effects, also promotes Th2 responses.

Evidence also exists that vitamin D plays an inhibitory role in Th2 responses. In a murine model of pulmonary eosinophilic inflammation, early treatment with vitamin D supported allergen-induced T-cell proliferation along with IL-4, IL-13, and immunoglobulin E production. However, the bronchoalveolar lavage fluid and lung tissue had impaired recruitment of eosinophils and low levels of IL-5.[36] A study by Pichler and colleagues[37] looked at the effects of 1,25-dihydroxyvitamin D on naive CD4$^+$ T helper and CD8$^+$ cytotoxic T cells from human cord cell cultures. They found that 1,25-dihydroxyvitamin D had inhibitory effects in the naive cells on IFN-γ production induced by IL-12, as well as IL-4 and IL-13 production induced by IL-4. This would suggest that vitamin D also helps blunt the Th2 response. Whether or not vitamin D favors a shift in the helper T cell balance toward Th1 versus Th2 dominance remains unclear. These variable results may be secondary to differences in the absolute amount of vitamin D exposure, the baseline vitamin D status (deficiency vs insufficiency vs sufficiency), and the timing of exposure (naive vs mature cell lines). More likely, at pharmacologic levels, vitamin D may inhibit Th1 and Th2 cell activation. Whether these known immune effects have translated into significant relationships between vitamin D levels and allergies, asthma, and atopic dermatitis is discussed later.

VITAMIN D AND ALLERGY

Several large birth cohort studies have examined the relationship between infant vitamin D supplementation and subsequent development of allergy and asthma. One study looked at a segment of the Northern Finland Birth Cohort from 1966 in which infants were given vitamin D supplements in the first year of life. Mothers reported the frequency and dose of vitamin D supplementation and the daily dose of vitamin D was calculated based on this information. Eighty-three percent of the subjects received 50 μg/d (2000 IU/d) of vitamin D.[38] Subjects received several follow-ups, including at 31 years of age at which the presence of asthma and atopy was assessed. After adjustment for social factors, the prevalence of atopy and allergic rhinitis at age 31 years was higher in subjects who received vitamin D supplementation as infants.[38] Another prospective birth cohort of more than 4000 infants 98% of whom were given supplements of vitamin A and D (400 IU/d of vitamin D) in either a water-soluble or peanut oil form showed that infants who received water-soluble supplements had a greater risk of asthma, food hypersensitivity, and aeroallergen sensitization at age 4 years than infants given peanut oil–based supplements.[39] No significant associations were seen for eczema or allergic rhinitis.[39] However, additional prospective work looking at maternal vitamin D dietary intake during pregnancy by Camargo and colleagues[23] showed that women in the highest quartile of vitamin D intake had a lower risk of having a child with recurrent wheeze at 3 years of age. These results may indicate that the timing of intervention in vitamin D levels may factor in subsequent allergic disease. An alternative explanation is that different absolute amounts of vitamin D have alternate physiologic effects on allergic pathogenesis. Furthermore, although beyond the scope of this review, vitamin D may also affect the body's susceptibility and response to infectious organisms, a major trigger of wheezing at a young age. The topic of vitamin D and infection in the setting of asthma has been reviewed elsewhere.[40]

Several surrogate markers of vitamin D deficiency have been evaluated in the context of allergy and asthma prevalence. People living at higher latitudes are known to be at greater risk for vitamin D deficiency.[24] A review of 166 pediatric cases of clinical rickets from 1986 to 2003 commented that in the 5 studies involving rickets in white children, all involved subjects were from northern states.[41] People who live at northern latitudes higher than 35° are unable to synthesize vitamin D from November to February.[8] Given the variations in latitude in the United States that may contribute to differences in sun exposure, the potential exists to compare populations in various geographic environments with respect to allergic disease. An exploratory study on surrogate markers for vitamin D and EpiPen/EpiPen Jr (Dey, Napa, CA, USA) prescriptions revealed that states in the New England region had a higher prescription rate than southern states after controlling for socioeconmic factors.[42] A surrogate marker of sunshine exposure, melanoma incidence, was inversely correlated with the EpiPen prescription rate, although average temperature and average precipitation were not.[42] An inverse relationship exists between body mass index and vitamin D status secondary to decreased bioavailability.[8] Prevalence of allergic disease in patients who underwent routine vitamin D screening as part of their care at an obesity clinic showed no association between vitamin D status and the prevalence of asthma or allergic rhinitis.[43] However, patients with vitamin D deficiency were more likely to report atopic dermatitis.[43]

VITAMIN D AND ASTHMA

Of the different disorders associated with allergic inflammation, perhaps asthma has been the most closely examined in the context of vitamin D. Consistent with earlier sections, evidence exists in support and against vitamin D deficiency contributing to the asthma epidemic. Extensive reviews of both sides of the argument have been published previously.[19,44]

Experimental models of asthma have been used to help test the vitamin D hypothesis. As mentioned previously, vitamin D has been shown in a murine model of eosinophilic inflammation to induce impaired recruitment of eosinophils and reduce levels of IL-5.[36] Data are also emerging that vitamin D affects glucocorticoid signaling pathyways. Xystrakis and colleagues[45] reported that the addition of vitamin D and dexamethasone to cultures of CD4+ T regulatory cells from steroid-resistant asthmatics enhanced IL-10 secretion from these cells to levels comparable with cells of steroid-sensitive patients treated with dexamethasone alone. Zhang and colleagues[46] have also reported that vitamin D enhances dexamethasone-induced mitogen-activated protein (MAP) kinase phosphatase-1 (MKP-1) expression in PBMCs, a pathway by which glucocorticoids exert their antiinflammatory effects. In patients referred to our institution with asthma, we have noted that serum vitamin D levels are inversely correlated with corticosteroid usage.[14] These laboratory and clinical observations raise the question of vitamin D supplementation potentially having a steroid-sparing effect in asthma.

Although the studies mentioned in the previous paragraph suggest a supportive role for vitamin D in asthma control, some experiments in KO mice do not support this association. Experimental allergic asthma induction was performed by Wittke and colleagues[47] in VDR KO and WT mice. The WT mice developed asthma, as expected. However, VDR KO mice failed to develop asthma after allergen induction. The administration of 1,25-dihydroxyvitamin D to WT mice had no effect on asthma severity, but did increase expression of 2 Th2-related genes. Some studies have described an association between VDR genetic polymorphisms and asthma, but this has not been replicated in subsequent experiments.[19]

Several clinical studies exist supporting a relationship between vitamin D status and asthma (**Table 2**). An analysis of more than 14,000 patients aged 20 years and using the NHANES database between 1988 and 1994 showed that subjects whose vitamin D level was in the highest quintile had significantly higher forced expiratory flow in first second of expiration (FEV_1) and forced vital capacity (FVC).[48] A recent paper on children with asthma from Costa Rica showed a significant association between

Table 2
Summary data on vitamin D and asthma and/or recurrent wheeze

Investigator	Population Studied	Results	References
Black and Scragg	>14,000 adults using the NHANES database	↑ FEV_1 and ↑ FVC in subjects whose vitamin D level was in the highest quintile	48
Brehm et al	Asthmatic children from Costa Rica	Log_{10} ↑ in vitamin D level associated with ↓ hospitalizations, ↓ antiinflammatory medication, and ↓ markers of allergy	49
Camargo et al	Mother-child prebirth cohort	Mothers in highest quartile of vitamin D intake had lower risk for child at age 3 years with recurrent wheeze	23
Devereux et al	Mother-child prebirth cohort	Mothers in highest quintile of vitamin D intake had lower risk for child at age 5 years to have ever wheezed, wheezing in the previous year, and persistent wheezing. No association of vitamin D levels with asthma, spirometry, or atopic sensitization	50
Gale et al	Mother-child prebirth cohort	Maternal 25-hydroxyvitamin D concentrations >30 ng/mL associated with an ↑ risk of eczema at 9 months and ↑ risk of asthma at 9 years	51

increasing vitamin D levels and reduced use of antiinflammatory medication in the previous year.[49]

Conflicting data exist on the influence of maternal vitamin D status and subsequent development of asthma. As mentioned previously, maternal intake of vitamin D has been associated with lower prevalence of wheezing at 3 years of age.[23] Another birth cohort from Scotland with information on maternal vitamin D intake had outcome measures analyzed at 5 years of age. The highest quintiles of maternal vitamin D intake were associated with reduced risk for ever wheezing, wheezing in the previous year, and persistent wheezing at ages 2 and 5 years.[50] Associations were independent of the children's vitamin D intake. Despite the wheezing associations, maternal vitamin D intake was not associated with asthma at age 5 years. In addition, maternal vitamin D intake was not associated with lower spirometry values or atopic sensitization.[50] A group of children from the United Kingdom were followed prospectively after vitamin D levels from their mothers were collected during pregnancy. The investigators found an increased risk of eczema at 9 months and asthma at 9 years in children whose mother's had a vitamin D level greater than 75 nmol/L (>30 ng/mL), although only 30% of patients were available for follow-up at 9 years.[51]

VITAMIN D AND ATOPIC DERMATITIS

Data have emerged regarding the molecular effects of vitamin D in the skin. VDR expression in the skin was first confirmed after rats injected with radiolabeled 1,25-dihydroxyvitamin D demonstrated radioactivity concentrated in the nuclei of the epidermis along with a variety of other tissues.[52] 1,25-Dihydroxyvitamin D has been shown to enhance keratinocyte differentiation, and have either stimulatory or suppressive effects on keratinocyte growth that is concentration dependent.[53] VDR expression on keratinocytes seems to be present only in proliferating cells and consequently, the basal keratinocyte is the main VDR-containing cell in the epidermis. Variable VDR expression based on the proliferating and differentiating state of the keratinocyte, as well as local cytokine-mediated interactions may provide an explanation for vitamin D's observed inhibitory effects in psoriatic skin and proliferative effects in normal skin.[53] Vitamin D has been shown to increase the synthesis of platelet-derived growth factor promoting wound healing, and tumor necrosis factor α promoting keratinocyte differentiation.[54,55] Decreased synthesis of IL-1α, IL-6, and RANTES secondary to vitamin D has resulted in decreased inflammation in epidermal keratinocytes.[56–58] The enzyme responsible for the initial hydroxylation of vitamin D to 25-hydroxyvitamin D and the enzyme responsible for the conversion of 25-hydroxyvitamin D into active 1,25-dihydroxyvitamin D (CYP27B1) are found in keratinocytes.[59] Vitamin D has also been shown to have a beneficial effect on the permeability barrier in the epidermis. Bikle and colleagues[60] studied mice null for the expression of CYP27B1. Lower levels of multiple proteins necessary for formation of the stratum corneum, including filaggrin, were lower in the null mice compared with the WT controls. Following tape disruption, null mice had a significantly delayed barrier recovery compared with WT mice.[60]

As mentioned previously, VDRs are located on macrophages and DCs, as is CYP27B1. 1,25-dihydroxyvitamin D has been shown to have inhibitory effects on the differentiation of DCs.[28] In vitro treatment of DCs with vitamin D leads to decreased IL-12 and enhanced IL-10. These cytokine effects, along with inhibitory effects on DC maturation, promote tolerogenic properties and suppressor T-cell induction.[28] A short treatment course of 1,25-dihydroxyvitamin D in mice induced tolerogenic DCs and increased T regulatory cells.[61]

The pathogenesis of atopic dermatitis involves epidermal barrier and immunologic dysfunction. Atopic dermatitis patients can have defects of the permeability barrier and the antimicrobial barrier of the stratum corneum.[62] The permeability barrier consists of hydrophobic lipids that percolate the extracellular environment of the stratum cornuem and prevent water loss into the outside environment.[62] Overactivity of serine proteases secondary to genetic defects, such as filaggrin and environmental stimuli, such as alkaline soaps, promotes reduction of hydration and extracellular lipids in the stratum corneum, introduction of antigens, and promotion of inflammation.[62] Loss of function mutations in the gene encoding filaggrin (FLG, located on chromosome 1q21 in a locus termed the epidermal differentiation complex) are associated with atopic dermatitis.[63] Population-based studies in European children show a threefold increased risk for atopic dermatitis in subjects with FLG variants and 18% to 48% of patients with atopic dermatitis carry an FLG null allele.[64]

Antimicrobial peptides (AMPs) are an important part of the antimicrobial barrier. AMPs are secreted on the surface of the skin as a first-line defense against infection. The release of AMPs can be triggered by toll-like receptors (TLRs). AMPs are secreted by many different cells in the skin, including keratinocytes and mast cells. Aside from their antimicrobial properties, they are believed to play a role in immune system signaling.[65] Cathelicidin is one of the most well known AMPs. Cathelicidin deficiency in the skin is known to be associated with atopic dermatitis. Ong and colleagues[66] reported significantly decreased immunostaining for cathelicidins in acute and chronic atopic dermatitis lesions compared with psoriatic skin lesions. This finding supports the differences in skin infections between patients with these 2 diseases. Amongst patients with atopic dermatitis, those with a history of herpes simplex virus (HSV) superinfection have significantly lower cathelicidin levels.[67] Antiviral assays have shown that cathelicidin has activity against HSV.[67] Skin from cathelicidin deficient mice has also been shown to have reduced ability to limit vaccinia virus proliferation.[68] A mulitcenter study to determine phenotypes associated with eczema herpeticum (ADEH) showed that patients with ADEH were more likely to experience cutaneous skin infections and have more Th2-polarized disease.[69]

Vitamin D has been shown to have a significant role in cathelicidin expression in the skin.[65] Wang and colleagues[70] showed that promoters of cathelicidin and beta2 defensin (another AMP) genes contain consensus vitamin D response elements and that 1,25-dihydroxyvitamin D promotes antimicrobial peptide gene expression. Liu and colleagues[71] reported that activation of TLRs by *Mycobacterium tuberculosis*–derived lipopeptide resulted in increased expression of VDR and CYP27B1 (the enzyme responsible for conversion of vitamin D into the active form) causing cathelicidin induction. Therefore, it has been proposed that skin infection or injury leads to activation of CYP27B1 and up-regulated VDR expression, which in turn leads to increased production of activated vitamin D and antimicrobial peptides.[65,71]

Given the potential for vitamin D to suppress inflammatory responses, enhance antimicrobial peptide activity, and promote the integrity of the permeability barrier, supplementation provides a possible therapeutic intervention for a variety of skin disorders, including atopic dermatitis. In a sample of 14 patients with moderate to severe atopic dermatitis who received 4000 IU/d of vitamin D_3 for 21 days, biopsied lesional skin showed a significant increase in cathelicidin expression.[72] A double-blind randomized controlled trial in children with winter-related atopic dermatitis (primarily mild) was performed using a regimen of 1000 IU/d of vitamin D for 1 month during the winter. Five subjects received supplementation and 6 subjects received placebo. Baseline changes in global assessments of skin showed that the group treated with vitamin D had a significant improvement in baseline score compared with placebo.[73] Future trials involving larger sample sizes and longer treatment periods will be necessary to more fully assess vitamin D as a therapeutic strategy in atopic dermatitis.

SUMMARY

Data on vitamin D insufficiency are expanding to include evidence on its role in asthma, allergic disorders, and atopic dermatitis. In addition to its well-documented relationship with rickets and bone metabolism, vitamin D is now recognized as an immunomodulator. However, conflicting data exist with respect to the role of vitamin D in the pathogenesis of allergic diseases. Future research on vitamin D supplementation will help determine if the sunshine vitamin can serve as an adjuvant treatment of asthma and atopic dermatitis.

REFERENCES

1. Mohr SB. A brief history of vitamin D and cancer prevention. Ann Epidemiol 2009; 19(2):79–83.
2. Palm T. The geographical distribution and etiology of rickets. Practitioner 1890; 45(270–9):321–42.
3. Mozolowski W, Sniadecki J. On the cure of rickets. Nature 1939;143:121.
4. Mellanby T. The part played by an 'accessory factor' in the production of experimental rickets. J Physiol 1918;52:11–4.
5. McCollum EV, Simmonds N, Becker JE, et al. Studies on experimental rickets. XXI. An experimental demonstration of the existence of a vitamin which promotes calcium deposition. J Biol Chem 1922;53:293–312.
6. Windaus A, Schenck F, von Werder F. On the antirachitic active irradiation product from 7-dehydrocholesterol. Physiol Chem 1936;241:100–3.
7. Holick M. Vitamin D: the underappreciated D-lightful hormone that is important for skeletal and cellular health. Curr Opin Endocrinol Diabetes 2002;9(1):87–98.
8. Holick MF. Vitamin D deficiency. N Engl J Med 2007;357(3):266–81.
9. Godar DE, Wengraitis SP, Shreffler J, et al. UV doses of Americans. Photochem Photobiol 2001;73(6):621–9.
10. Godar DE. UV doses of American children and adolescents. Photochem Photobiol 2001;74(6):787–93.
11. Ginde AA, Liu MC, Camargo CA Jr. Demographic differences and trends of vitamin D insufficiency in the US population, 1988–2004. Arch Intern Med 2009; 169(6):626–32.
12. Kumar J, Muntner P, Kaskel FJ, et al. Prevalence and associations of 25-hydroxyvitamin D deficiency in US children: NHANES 2001–2004. Pediatrics 2009;124:e362–70.
13. NHANES. Analytical note for NHANES 2000–2006 and NHANES III (1988–1994) 25-hydroxyvitamin D analysis. 2009. Available at: www.cdc.gov/nchs/data/nhanes/nhanes3/VitaminD_analyticnote.pdf. Accessed September 25, 2009.
14. Searing DA, Murphy J, Hauk P, et al. Vitamin D levels in children with asthma, atopic dermatitis, and food allergy. J Allergy Clin Immunol 2010;125(2):AB44.
15. Wagner CL, Greer FR. Prevention of rickets and vitamin D deficiency in infants, children, and adolescents. Pediatrics 2008;122(5):1142–52.
16. NIH. Dietary supplement fact sheet: vitamin D. 2009. Available at: http://dietary-supplements.info.nih.gov/factsheets/vitamind.asp#h3. Accessed October 25, 2009.
17. Vieth R, Bischoff-Ferrari H, Boucher BJ, et al. The urgent need to recommend an intake of vitamin D that is effective. Am J Clin Nutr 2007;85(3):649–50.

18. Barger-Lux MJ, Heaney RP, Dowell S, et al. Vitamin D and its major metabolites: serum levels after graded oral dosing in healthy men. Osteoporos Int 1998;8(3):222–30.
19. Litonjua AA, Weiss ST. Is vitamin D deficiency to blame for the asthma epidemic? J Allergy Clin Immunol 2007;120(5):1031–5.
20. Asher M. Worldwide variations in the prevalence of asthma symptoms: the International Study of Asthma and Allergies in Childhood (ISAAC). Eur Respir J 1998; 12(2):315–35.
21. Von Mutius E. Epidemiology of allergic disease. In: Leung DYM, Sampson HA, Geha RS, et al, editors. Pediatric allergy principles and practice. St. Louis (MO): Mosby; 2003. p. 1–9.
22. Zhao T, Wang HJ, Chen Y, et al. Prevalence of childhood asthma, allergic rhinitis and eczema in Urumqi and Beijing. J Paediatr Child Health 2000;36(2):128–33.
23. Camargo CA Jr, Rifas-Shiman SL, Litonjua AA, et al. Maternal intake of vitamin D during pregnancy and risk of recurrent wheeze in children at 3 y of age. Am J Clin Nutr 2007;85(3):788–95.
24. Misra M, Pacaud D, Petryk A, et al. Vitamin D deficiency in children and its management: review of current knowledge and recommendations. Pediatrics 2008;122(2):398–417.
25. Baker AR, McDonnell DP, Hughes M, et al. Cloning and expression of full-length cDNA encoding human vitamin D receptor. Proc Natl Acad Sci U S A 1988; 85(10):3294–8.
26. Bhalla AK, Amento EP, Clemens TL, et al. Specific high-affinity receptors for 1,25-dihydroxyvitamin D3 in human peripheral blood mononuclear cells: presence in monocytes and induction in T lymphocytes following activation. J Clin Endocrinol Metab 1983;57(6):1308–10.
27. Brennan A, Katz DR, Nunn JD, et al. Dendritic cells from human tissues express receptors for the immunoregulatory vitamin D3 metabolite, dihydroxycholecalciferol. Immunology 1987;61(4):457–61.
28. Adorini L, Penna G, Giarratana N, et al. Dendritic cells as key targets for immunomodulation by vitamin D receptor ligands. J Steroid Biochem Mol Biol 2004; 89–90(1–5):437–41.
29. Adams JS, Gacad MA. Characterization of 1 alpha-hydroxylation of vitamin D3 sterols by cultured alveolar macrophages from patients with sarcoidosis. J Exp Med 1985;161(4):755–65.
30. Chen KS, DeLuca HF. Cloning of the human 1 alpha,25-dihydroxyvitamin D-3 24-hydroxylase gene promoter and identification of two vitamin D-responsive elements. Biochim Biophys Acta 1995;1263(1):1–9.
31. Provvedini DM, Tsoukas CD, Deftos LJ, et al. 1,25-Dihydroxyvitamin D3 receptors in human leukocytes. Science 1983;221(4616):1181–3.
32. Tsoukas CD, Provvedini DM, Manolagas SC. 1,25-Dihydroxyvitamin D3: a novel immunoregulatory hormone. Science 1984;224(4656):1438–40.
33. Mahon BD, Wittke A, Weaver V, et al. The targets of vitamin D depend on the differentiation and activation status of CD4 positive T cells. J Cell Biochem 2003;89(5):922–32.
34. Froicu M, Weaver V, Wynn TA, et al. A crucial role for the vitamin D receptor in experimental inflammatory bowel diseases. Mol Endocrinol 2003;17(12):2386–92.
35. Boonstra A, Barrat FJ, Crain C, et al. 1alpha, 25-Dihydroxyvitamin D3 has a direct effect on naive CD4(+) T cells to enhance the development of Th2 cells. J Immunol 2001;167(9):4974–80.
36. Matheu V, Back O, Mondoc E, et al. Dual effects of vitamin D-induced alteration of TH1/TH2 cytokine expression: enhancing IgE production and decreasing airway

eosinophilia in murine allergic airway disease. J Allergy Clin Immunol 2003; 112(3):585–92.

37. Pichler J, Gerstmayr M, Szepfalusi Z, et al. 1 alpha, 25(OH)$_2$D$_3$ inhibits not only Th1 but also Th2 differentiation in human cord blood T cells. Pediatr Res 2002; 52(1):12–8.

38. Hypponen E, Sovio U, Wjst M, et al. Infant vitamin D supplementation and allergic conditions in adulthood: northern Finland birth cohort 1966. Ann N Y Acad Sci 2004;1037:84–95.

39. Kull I, Bergstrom A, Melen E, et al. Early-life supplementation of vitamins A and D, in water-soluble form or in peanut oil, and allergic diseases during childhood. J Allergy Clin Immunol 2006;118(6):1299–304.

40. Ginde AA, Mansbach JM, Camargo CA Jr. Vitamin D, respiratory infections, and asthma. Curr Allergy Asthma Rep 2009;9(1):81–7.

41. Weisberg P, Scanlon KS, Li R, et al. Nutritional rickets among children in the United States: review of cases reported between 1986 and 2003. Am J Clin Nutr 2004;80(6 Suppl):1697S–705.

42. Camargo CA Jr, Clark S, Kaplan MS, et al. Regional differences in EpiPen prescriptions in the United States: the potential role of vitamin D. J Allergy Clin Immunol 2007;120(1):131–6.

43. Oren E, Banerji A, Camargo CA Jr. Vitamin D and atopic disorders in an obese population screened for vitamin D deficiency. J Allergy Clin Immunol 2008; 121(2):533–4.

44. Wjst M. The vitamin D slant on allergy. Pediatr Allergy Immunol 2006;17(7): 477–83.

45. Xystrakis E, Kusumakar S, Boswell S, et al. Reversing the defective induction of IL-10-secreting regulatory T cells in glucocorticoid-resistant asthma patients. J Clin Invest 2006;116(1):146–55.

46. Zhang Y, Goleva E, Leung DY. Vitamin D enhances glucocorticoid-induced mitogen-activated protein kinase phosphatase-1 (MKP-1) expression and their anti-proliferative effect in peripheral blood mononuclear cells. J Allergy Clin Immunol 2009;123(2):S121.

47. Wittke A, Weaver V, Mahon BD, et al. Vitamin D receptor-deficient mice fail to develop experimental allergic asthma. J Immunol 2004;173(5):3432–6.

48. Black PN, Scragg R. Relationship between serum 25-hydroxyvitamin D and pulmonary function in the Third National Health and Nutrition Examination Survey. Chest 2005;128(6):3792–8.

49. Brehm JM, Celedon JC, Soto-Quiros ME, et al. Serum vitamin D levels and markers of severity of childhood asthma in Costa Rica. Am J Respir Crit Care Med 2009;179(9):765–71.

50. Devereux G, Litonjua AA, Turner SW, et al. Maternal vitamin D intake during pregnancy and early childhood wheezing. Am J Clin Nutr 2007;85(3):853–9.

51. Gale CR, Robinson SM, Harvey NC, et al. Maternal vitamin D status during pregnancy and child outcomes. Eur J Clin Nutr 2008;62(1):68–77.

52. Stumpf WE, Sar M, Reid FA, et al. Target cells for 1,25-dihydroxyvitamin D3 in intestinal tract, stomach, kidney, skin, pituitary, and parathyroid. Science 1979; 206(4423):1188–90.

53. Gurlek A, Pittelkow MR, Kumar R. Modulation of growth factor/cytokine synthesis and signaling by 1alpha,25-dihydroxyvitamin D(3): implications in cell growth and differentiation. Endocr Rev 2002;23(6):763–86.

54. Zhang JZ, Maruyama K, Ono I, et al. Production and secretion of platelet-derived growth factor AB by cultured human keratinocytes: regulatory effects of phorbol

12-myristate 13-acetate, etretinate, 1,25-dihydroxyvitamin D3, and several cytokines. J Dermatol 1995;22(5):305–9.

55. Geilen CC, Bektas M, Wieder T, et al. 1alpha,25-dihydroxyvitamin D3 induces sphingomyelin hydrolysis in HaCaT cells via tumor necrosis factor alpha. J Biol Chem 1997;272(14):8997–9001.

56. Zhang JZ, Maruyama K, Ono I, et al. Regulatory effects of 1,25-dihydroxyvitamin D3 and a novel vitamin D3 analogue MC903 on secretion of interleukin-1 alpha (IL-1 alpha) and IL-8 by normal human keratinocytes and a human squamous cell carcinoma cell line (HSC-1). J Dermatol Sci 1994;7(1):24–31.

57. Komine M, Watabe Y, Shimaoka S, et al. The action of a novel vitamin D3 analogue, OCT, on immunomodulatory function of keratinocytes and lymphocytes. Arch Dermatol Res 1999;291(9):500–6.

58. Fukuoka M, Ogino Y, Sato H, et al. RANTES expression in psoriatic skin, and regulation of RANTES and IL-8 production in cultured epidermal keratinocytes by active vitamin D3 (tacalcitol). Br J Dermatol 1998;138(1):63–70.

59. Bikle DD, Chang S, Crumrine D, et al. 25-Hydroxyvitamin D 1 alpha-hydroxylase is required for optimal epidermal differentiation and permeability barrier homeostasis. J Invest Dermatol 2004;122(4):984–92.

60. Bikle DD, Pillai S, Gee E, et al. Regulation of 1,25-dihydroxyvitamin D production in human keratinocytes by interferon-gamma. Endocrinology 1989;124(2):655–60.

61. Gregori S, Casorati M, Amuchastegui S, et al. Regulatory T cells induced by 1 alpha,25-dihydroxyvitamin D3 and mycophenolate mofetil treatment mediate transplantation tolerance. J Immunol 2001;167(4):1945–53.

62. Elias PM, Hatano Y, Williams ML. Basis for the barrier abnormality in atopic dermatitis: outside-inside-outside pathogenic mechanisms. J Allergy Clin Immunol 2008;121(6):1337–43.

63. O'Regan GM, Sandilands A, McLean WH, et al. Filaggrin in atopic dermatitis. J Allergy Clin Immunol 2008;122(4):689–93.

64. Irvine AD. Fleshing out filaggrin phenotypes. J Invest Dermatol 2007;127(3):504–7.

65. Schauber J, Gallo RL. Antimicrobial peptides and the skin immune defense system. J Allergy Clin Immunol 2008;122(2):261–6.

66. Ong PY, Ohtake T, Brandt C, et al. Endogenous antimicrobial peptides and skin infections in atopic dermatitis. N Engl J Med 2002;347(15):1151–60.

67. Howell MD, Wollenberg A, Gallo RL, et al. Cathelicidin deficiency predisposes to eczema herpeticum. J Allergy Clin Immunol 2006;117(4):836–41.

68. Howell MD, Gallo RL, Boguniewicz M, et al. Cytokine milieu of atopic dermatitis skin subverts the innate immune response to vaccinia virus. Immunity 2006; 24(3):341–8.

69. Beck LA, Boguniewicz M, Hata T, et al. Phenotype of atopic dermatitis subjects with a history of eczema herpeticum. J Allergy Clin Immunol 2009;124(2):260–9.

70. Wang TT, Nestel FP, Bourdeau V, et al. Cutting edge: 1,25-dihydroxyvitamin D3 is a direct inducer of antimicrobial peptide gene expression. J Immunol 2004; 173(5):2909–12.

71. Liu PT, Stenger S, Li H, et al. Toll-like receptor triggering of a vitamin D-mediated human antimicrobial response. Science 2006;311(5768):1770–3.

72. Hata TR, Kotol P, Jackson M, et al. Administration of oral vitamin D induces cathelicidin production in atopic individuals. J Allergy Clin Immunol 2008;122(4): 829–31.

73. Sidbury R, Sullivan AF, Thadhani RI, et al. Randomized controlled trial of vitamin D supplementation for winter-related atopic dermatitis in Boston: a pilot study. Br J Dermatol 2008;159(1):245–7.

Complementary and Alternative Interventions in Atopic Dermatitis

Joohee Lee, MD[a], Leonard Bielory, MD[b,c,]*

KEYWORDS

- Complementary and alternative medicine • Atopic dermatitis
- Chinese herbal therapy • Herbal medicine
- Biologically based therapies

Ever since the 1997 landmark study by Eisenberg,[1] there has been a growing awareness of the prevalence of CAM use by the general population. In December 2008, the National Center for Complementary and Alternative Medicine (NCCAM) released updated findings regarding CAM use based on the 2007 National Health Interview Survey. Of the 23,393 adults older than 18 years and 9417 children younger than 17 years, approximately 38% of adults and approximately 12% of children in the United States use some form of CAM (http://nccam.nih.gov/news/camstats.htm). The 2007 National Health Statistics Report has identified the use of a common group of nonvitamin, nonmineral natural products for therapy (17.7% of all CAM use) (http://nccam.nih.gov/news/2008/nhsr12.pdf).

A wide range of herbal products is available to the consumer/patient with allergic diseases. About 15 years ago, the herbal industry was in essence deregulated by the passage of the congressional Dietary Supplement Health and Education Act of 1994, which restricted the role of the US Food and Drug Administration in classifying herbal products.[2] Critical reviews of the available literature on herbal medicines have concluded that published data on the therapeutic effects of herbals on allergic

Financial disclosures: J. Lee, none; L. Bielory: Schering-Plough, Glaxo-Smith-Kline, Merck, Otsuka, Novartis, Sanofi-Aventis, Genentech, Astellas, UCB-Pharma, Alcon, Meda, Inspire, Santen, Allergan, ISTA, SARCode, Bausch & Lomb, Vistakon, ViroPharm, Dyax, Jerini, Ocusense (Tear Lab), Rutgers University Press
a Department of Internal Medicine, Mayo Clinic, 200 First Street South West, Rochester, MN 55905, USA
b Rutgers University, Center for Environmental Prediction, 14 College Farm Road, New Brunswick, NJ 08901-8551, USA
c STARx Allergy and Asthma Center, 400 Mountain Avenue, Springfield, NJ 07081-2515, USA
* Corresponding author. STARx Allergy and Asthma Center, 400 Mountain Avenue, Springfield, NJ 07081-2515.
E-mail address: drbielory@gmail.com

Immunol Allergy Clin N Am 30 (2010) 411–424
doi:10.1016/j.iac.2010.06.006
0889-8561/10/$ – see front matter © 2010 Published by Elsevier Inc.
immunology.theclinics.com

diseases are conflicting and riddled with deficiencies in quality of design.[3,4] However, for the clinician, it is important to recognize that consumption of CAM interventions continues to thrive despite the lack of strong clinical evidence of efficacy. Epidemiologic data indicate that the use of complementary interventions is common in atopic disorders, especially atopic dermatitis (AD), allergic rhinitis, and asthma.[5] In a study performed in Scandinavia, 227 of 444 (51.1%) patients with AD reported previous or current use of one or more forms of complementary interventions. The most common forms were homeopathy, health-food preparations, and herbal remedies.[6] In a 2007 survey of alternative medicine use in AD, it was found that herbal remedies and homeopathic products were given by parents of 34 of 80 pediatric patients with AD.[7]

The above-mentioned epidemiologic studies have identified motivating factors for CAM use. Among adults, disease duration, severity of the disease, and the perceived ineffective treatment of standard therapy were cited as common reasons for trying CAM interventions. In pediatric patients, parents commonly tried specific interventions based on recommendation from others (47%). A fear of steroid side effects (26.4%) and dissatisfaction with conventional treatment (17.6%) were also common driving factors.[7] For the clinician, such data emphasize the importance of careful medication history-taking, easing fears regarding topical steroids by educating patients and caregivers, and making sure that conventional treatments are used appropriately.[8]

In the aforementioned survey of the parents of 80 patients with AD, most alternative treatments were perceived to have no therapeutic effect, and clinical worsening of AD was reported in 2 instances.[7] There are several reported adverse effects associated with CAM use, which makes a strong case for the importance of a more systematic approach for establishing and maintaining patient-physician dialogue on both allopathic and alternative therapeutics. Of great concern are the potentially serious organ-specific side effects from alternative therapies for AD, including death, published in case reports. Other adverse effects include severe bilateral cataract formation in an 11-year-old boy after 8 months of treatment with an unidentified herbal medicine, although he had normal results on ophthalmologic examination 1 year before presentation.[9] Lenses of both eyes had severe posterior subcapsular and posterior capsular opacification. Correction of visual acuity was achieved after extensive surgery and lens implantation. Severe cardiomyopathy has been reported in association with a 2-week course of Chinese herbal medicine.[10] The connection between the 2 conditions was not made until 2 weeks after presentation when the patient was specifically asked if she had ingested any unusual substances. A review article of the potential harms of herbal medicines used for AD identified arsenic- and mercury-containing remedies that can produce eczematous lesions.[11] This article offers helpful tables delineating the various dermatoses reported in association with a wide range of popular herbal remedies, including kava, aloe vera, as well as adulterated therapeutic products.

Population-based research regarding CAM use for allergic diseases underscores the increasing challenge for health care providers with respect to identifying CAM use and ensuring safe use of allopathic and complementary medicines in disease management. A recent review by Engler and colleagues[12] provides a timely overview on this topic, proposing a practical 10-step approach to establishing patient-physician cooperation with regards to CAM use. Furthermore, Engler and colleagues acknowledge the challenge of synthesizing available data on specific alternative therapies and they identify 2 trustworthy and active databases for physicians and specialists. One is the website of the NCCAM branch of the National Institutes of Health (http://nccam. nih.gov/), which provides data formatted for patients and physicians. In addition, the Natural Medicines Comprehensive Database (http://www.naturaldatabase.com) offers practical assessments of the research behind almost 1100 natural ingredients and more than 30,000 commercially available brand name products. It accounts for key quality markers such as randomization, allocation concealment, adequate blinding, and other factors using the principles from the Cochrane Collaboration. Furthermore, the database is regularly maintained and updated. It serves as a valuable tool for the clinician, as it integrates not only grading of efficacy but also that of safety and product quality/purity from international regulatory bodies.

Because of the lack of regulation, there is valid concern regarding the active ingredients in "natural" topical preparations, specifically potent corticosteroids. A study by Ramsay and colleagues[13] found that the majority of effective herbal creams used by 19 pediatric patients contained potent steroids, as detected by high-performance liquid chromatography. The most common steroid was high-potency clobetasol proprionate, which was found in 5 creams labeled Wau Wa and Muijiza. The remaining herbal creams contained clobetasol proprionate and hydrocortisone, betamethasone valerate, clobetasone butyrate, and hydrocortisone. Parents were not aware that the creams contained steroids.[13]

Epidemiologic data have been stimuli for better elucidation of the efficacy of CAM interventions for allergic diseases. Despite the concern of the harms and risks associated with the use of alternative therapies, the research in this area continues to grow and offers some promising avenues for these frustrating and increasingly prevalent conditions. There have been hundreds of clinical trials looking at the effect of CAM on asthma, allergic rhinitis, and AD. Mainardi and colleagues[4] have reviewed recent studies that have taken on a more sophisticated focus on mechanistic biochemical pathways of signal transduction and transcription of T-cell effectors and mediators by which anti-allergic effects of various nonconventional medicines might be achieved. The following discussion of complementary and alternative interventions that have been studied for AD treatment has been organized to reflect the classification system endorsed by NCCAM.

BIOLOGY-BASED PRACTICES
Probiotics

The intestinal microbiota plays an important role in immune development and may play a role in the development of allergic disorders. According to the revised hygiene hypothesis, the increase in prevalence of atopic diseases over the past several decades is considered as the immunologic consequence of a changed intestinal colonization pattern in infants. The microorganisms comprising endogenous flora of the normal gastrointestinal tract are believed to play a role in "educating" the neonate's immune system. This education includes converting the T_H2-biased prenatal responses into "balanced immune responses," which include tolerance to self-antigens and promoting the maturation of immune responses in other tissues.[14,15]

There is increasing interest in the use of probiotics (live beneficial microorganisms, primarily of the Lactobacillus and Bifidobacteria genus, characteristic of the healthy infant gut microbiota) and prebiotics (nondigestible oligosaccharides that promote the selective growth of nonpathogenic strains of commensal bacteria), used alone or together (synbiotics), to influence intestinal microbiota and modulate immune responses in vitro and in vivo.[16] It is not entirely surprising that promising observations at the bench have not neatly translated to benefit at the bedside. The landmark study by Kalliomaki and colleagues[17] was the first report that the frequency of AD in neonates treated with Lactobacillus rhamnosus GG was half that of the placebo.

Sustained prevention was seen at 4 years out.[18] However, numerous trials using strains of *Lactobacillus* reported negative results, with no difference in the development of AD between the intervention and placebo arms.[19–21] It is worth noting that the study designs of these trials with negative results were not identical to those of the Kalliomaki study (prenatal and postnatal supplementation), as 2 of these trials started probiotic supplementation postnatally.

The heterogeneity of study design found among trials of prebiotics and probiotics poses a challenge to data synthesis. A recent review of randomized controlled trials of probiotics for AD reviewed 7 prevention studies and 12 treatment studies and found that overall results were conflicting.[22] At present, there is not enough evidence to support the use of pro-, pre- or synbiotics for prevention or treatment of AD in children in clinical practice.[23] Furthermore, 2 trials in particular have raised the question of whether or not there may be a more insidious effect of predisposing children to developing allergic respiratory diseases with use.[19,20]

It would be premature to dismiss the therapeutic potential of pro-, pre-, or synbiotics. Numerous review articles have suggested that the following details need to be addressed: (1) effective bacterial species/strains, (2) optimal dosing, (3) whether there is added benefit with synbiotics, (4) the optimal timing for intervention, and (5) the patient populations that would gain the most benefit.[22,24] Effects may vary depending on the characteristics of the study population, such as whether the infant was delivered by caesarean section, and in the case of AD associated with elevated IgE.[25,26] The same point can also be made when considering the limited study of prebiotics for AD prevention. One study found a significant reduction in the incidence of AD in infants who were at risk for developing AD.[27] Another study observed a higher incidence of AD associated with prebiotic use, but this study looked at formula-fed healthy infants.[28] In terms of AD treatment, a beneficial effect of probiotics has been observed in a trial of children with more severe AD.[29]

A search of the literature revealed 1 article in a German publication that reviews ongoing research on topical preparations of probiotics, which is an intriguing notion to consider in light of our dominant medical paradigm of antibiotics.[30] It will be interesting to see if and how this approach will play a role in AD therapy.

Vitamin B_{12}

Use of vitamin B_{12} in allergy is not a new therapeutic concept. However, in the past 10 years, in vitro investigation of inflammatory dermatoses, including AD, has drawn attention to the pathophysiologic role of overexpression of inducible nitric oxide synthase (iNOS). Lesional skin (upper dermal microvasculature) from AD has been demonstrated to have an increased expression of iNOS.[31] Moreover, serum nitrate levels in Japanese children with AD have been shown to increase as compared with nonatopic controls and were found to correlate with disease severity and peripheral eosinophil counts.[32] The reduction of pruritus and erythema observed in 15 patients with AD who were given a topical nitric oxide synthase inhibitor[33] inspired one group of German investigators to focus on vitamin B_{12} on the basis of its ability to inactivate nitric oxide. In their prospective placebo-controlled randomized clinical trial of 41 adults with AD, topical vitamin B_{12} was shown to be superior to placebo with respect to reducing the extent and severity of AD as assessed by the Modified Six Area Six Sign Atopic Dermatitis score.[34] In this trial, each patient applied the vitamin B_{12}–containing cream to lesions on one side of the body and the placebo preparation on lesions on the contralateral side. However, a fair amount of cutaneous reactions were reported, including AD flare and local irritation.

Vitamin D

A role for vitamin D in atopic diseases including AD has been the subject of a growing number of studies (see the article by Searing and Leung elsewhere in this issue for further exploration of this topic). Recently, lack of vitamin D has been proposed as one of several environmental factors responsible for the increase in atopic diseases. Studies of maternal dietary intake of vitamin D have noted a lower frequency of atopic disease in the children of mothers with higher intake.[35] Conversely, a birth cohort study of 123 children sought to determine whether the estimated dose of dietary vitamin D_3 (recorded in a previous study) during the first year of life was associated with atopic diseases up to the age of 6 years, as determined by questionnaire-based survey.[36] Atopic manifestations were more prevalent in the group with higher intake of vitamin D_3. As more data are gathered, vitamin D supplementation may have a place in AD prevention in the prenatal period, whereas in the postnatal period, modified or limited vitamin D_3 supplementation will be necessary.

MAS063DP

MAS063DP (Atopiclair) is an emollient preparation that contains the active metabolite of *Glycyrrhiza glabra* (licorice) and *Vitis vinifera* (grapevine), a potential antioxidant. It has been recently approved for mild to moderate AD.[37] The efficacy of MAS063DP was established by a multicenter trial that looked at 60 pediatric patients (between ages 2 and 17 years) with mild to moderate AD treated for 6 weeks, with clinical evaluations at baseline and at days 8, 15, 22, 29, and 43. MAS063DP was associated with a statistically significant reduction in AD severity score at day 22 compared with vehicle. A statistically significant difference was sustained until the end of the study.[38]

AOA

Severe AD can be associated with cataract formation. One Japanese group published the findings from clinical application of an oral antioxidant, named AOA, derived from numerous seeds (eg, soybean, sesame, wheat germ). The extract was heated with infrared rays (4–14 μm wavelength), fermented with *Aspergillus oryzae*, and lipophilized with similarly heated sesame oil. This processing has been demonstrated to release low–molecular-weight antioxidants that are active and more bioavailable. Approximately half the patients with cataract-associated AD tested showed marked improvement.[39] An Internet search indicates that AOA has been evaluated in clinical use for AD as a topical preparation that also includes low levels of corticosteroids.

γ-LINOLENIC ACID

Evening primrose (*Oenothera biennis*) has been reported to have a potential benefit in AD, a property that is now linked to the plant's high content of γ-linolenic acid (GLA) as well as omega-6 fatty acids.[40] The immunologic basis for this property may be related to an abnormality in fatty acid metabolism in AD. The postulation is that atopic patients may have a deficiency in GLA, which is a precursor of prostaglandin E_1, an important component in normal T lymphocyte function.[40] Preliminary results of supplementation with 500 mg of evening primrose oil (EPO) containing 45 mg of GLA included data from 46 adults and 20 children. A subsequent report described improvement of itch with low-dose EPO and a 43% reduction in AD severity among the adults.[41] However, other trials have reported negative findings[42–44] as well as positive effects.[45,46] Overall, the body of evidence for EPO has been evaluated to be rather weak, and it cannot be endorsed as an effective treatment.[47]

Borage oil is another herbal agent with high GLA content that has been studied for treatment and prevention of AD. Published trials have evaluated therapy in adults and children. Adults were given 920 mg γ-linolenic acid, and children, 460 mg twice daily for 12 weeks. No significant benefit was noted with supplementation.[48] A later trial looked at supplementation with higher levels of GLA. Although it did not report statistically significant differences in therapeutic effect, significant differences favoring borage oil were observed when individuals who failed to show an increase in a serum surrogate marker and who were suspected of noncompliance were excluded from analysis.[43] Oral supplementation with 100 mg of GLA failed to show preventive benefit at 1 year of age in formula-fed infants with maternal history of atopic disease. However, GLA supplementation did show a favorable trend for AD severity. An increase in GLA concentrations in plasma phospholipids between baseline and 3 months of age was negatively associated with the severity of AD at 1 year.[49]

ST JOHN'S WORT

Hyperforin, identified as a major component of St John's wort (*Hypericum perforatum*), has antiinflammatory and antibacterial properties. This herbal extract, standardized to a 1.5% hyperforin (verum) preparation, has been studied in 21 individuals with mild to moderate AD in a one-sided comparison study with an emollient vehicle. Eighteen patients completed the 4-week treatment period. Primary outcome was AD severity, determined by a modified Scoring Atopic Dermatitis (SCORAD) index. The intensity of the eczematous lesions improved with the intervention and with the placebo. Although the intervention was significantly superior to the vehicle at all clinical visits ($P<.05$), it is unknown how this compares with topical corticosteroids.[50]

PERSIMMON LEAF EXTRACT

In vitro and in vivo studies have been published on the effects of persimmon leaf extract, which contains elements, including astragalin, that have been shown to inhibit histamine release by the human basophil cell line KU812 in response to cross-linkage of high-affinity IgE receptors.[51] Oral intake of both persimmon leaf and astragalin in mice attenuated passive cutaneous reactions and suppressed scratching behavior and elevation of serum IgE levels. Histologic analyses revealed significant reduction in inflammation and transepidermal water loss.[51,52]

BAMBOO STEM EXTRACT

Bambusae caulis in Liquamen (BCL) is a nutritious liquid extracted from heat-treated fresh bamboo stems, an herbal medicine that has been used to treat cough and asthma in East Asia. One group evaluated the antiinflammatory, antiallergenic, and immunoregulating properties of this extract in a murine model of 2,4-dinitrochlorobenzene–induced AD-like skin lesions in hairless mice.[53] BCL extract applied to the lesions inhibited the development of these lesions, with lower numbers of infiltrating leukocytes. BCL administration was also associated with suppression of serum IgE levels, attenuation of messenger RNA (mRNA) expression of interleukin (IL)-4, IL-13, and tumor necrosis factor (TNF) α, and induction of interferon (IFN)-γ expression in the spleen.[53]

SYNERGY BETWEEN PROBIOTICS AND HERBAL MEDICINE?

A recent study presents an interesting concept of probiotic-fermented herbal medicine.[54] Select herbal extracts were fermented in *Lactobacillus plantarum* (FHE) for anti-AD effects. The effects of FHE were evaluated using a murine model of AD induced by dust mite extract. The fermentation was demonstrated to increase bioavailability, and the end product exerted a dose-dependent inhibition of mitogen-induced splenic T- and B-lymphocyte proliferation. A reduction in plasma levels of IgE was also noted. Analysis of cytokine mRNA expression demonstrated suppression that was comparable to that seen with cyclosporine. Therefore, probiotic fermentation may have therapeutic advantages of increasing the bioavailability and immunosuppressive properties of herbal medicines.[54]

WHOLE MEDICAL SYSTEMS

All of the published trials in this area of alternative medicine (eg, traditional Chinese medicine, Kampo) used herbal combinations. Much of the benefit observed with the following herbal medications has been as an adjunctive, as opposed to an alternative therapy.

Clinical Trials

Overall, there are few randomized controlled trials of Chinese herbal therapy with sufficient powering. A 1999 double-blind, placebo-controlled, crossover trial with 40 adult patients with recalcitrant AD looked at the efficacy of Zemaphyte, a Chinese herbal oral preparation containing licorice, along with 9 other herbs commonly used for treatment of AD.[55] A 2005 update of a Cochrane review of traditional Chinese herbal mixtures identified 4 randomized controlled trials (159 individuals aged 1 to 60 years), all looking at the proprietary herbal mixture Zemaphyte (no longer being manufactured), that met the inclusion criteria.[56] Three of these trials used crossover design, and reduction of erythema and surface damage was greater with Zemaphyte than with placebo in 2 of these studies. Quality of sleep was higher in the treatment arm. The fourth trial was an open-label study comparing Zemaphyte in 2 different forms. There was a reduction in erythema and surface damage with both formulations, but no comparison between the 2 formulations was reported. Some adverse effects were reported in all 4 trials, but none were regarded as serious.[56] Overall, the studies had poor reporting and results were heterogeneous. The withdrawal rates ranged from 7.5% to 22.5%, and no trial used intention to treat analysis.

PentaHerbs is a formulation of 5 herbs (Cortex Moutan, root bark of Paeonia suffruticosa Andr (Ranunculaceae), Cortex Phellodendri, bark of Phellodendron chinensis Schneid (Rutaceae), Flos Lonicerae, flower of Lonicera japonica Thunb (Caprifoliaceae), Herba Menthae, aerial part of Mentha haplocalyx Briq (Labiatae), and Rhizoma Atractylodis, rhizome of Atractylodes lancea (Thunb) DC; 2:2:2:1:2 composition) that has been under investigation for several years. The initial trial in 2004 was an open-label study and enrolled 9 children, treated for 4 months.[57] In a confirmatory study, the medication was verified to be free of steroids (hydrocortisone, prednisolone, fludrocortisone, and dexamethasone) by thin-layer chromatography, infrared spectrophotometry, and liquid chromatography mass spectrometry.[58] In 2007, this same group published the findings of the use of the 5 herbal ingredients (PentaHerbs formulation, PHF) in a randomized and placebo-controlled clinical trial of 87 children with moderate to severe AD.[59] Twice-daily PHF reduced topical corticosteroid use and improved the quality of life in children with moderate to severe AD. The adverse reaction profiles seen among these patients were comparable with those observed in the placebo group, most common effects being upper respiratory infections ($P = .828$), diarrhea ($P = .074$), and abdominal pain ($P = .381$).[59]

Additional publications by this group focused on observable immunomodulatory effects to account for clinical benefit. Twenty-eight children with AD were treated with PHF for 3 months, and their mean plasma concentrations of inflammatory mediators, brain-derived neurotrophic factor (BDNF), and thymus and activation-regulated chemokine (TARC) decreased significantly from 1798 and 824 pg/mL at baseline to 1378 and 492 pg/mL ($P = .002$ and .013, respectively) at study completion.[60] Cell cultures showed dose-dependent suppression of peripheral blood mononuclear cell (PBMC) proliferation, reduction of supernatant concentrations of BDNF, IFN-γ, and TNF-α in response to PHA, and reduction in levels of BDNF and TARC following staphylococcus enterotoxin B stimulation. At the mRNA level, PHF suppressed the transcription of BDNF, TARC, IFN-γ, and TNF-α.[60] PHF and 2 of its 5 components were also observed to significantly reduce histamine release and prostaglandin D_2 synthesis in rat peritoneal mast cells activated by anti-IgE and compound 48/80 ($P<.05$).[61]

A small-scale prospective uncontrolled trial examined the therapeutic benefits of acupuncture combined with Chinese herbal medicine.[62] Twenty individuals aged between 13 and 48 years with mild to severe AD were treated with a 12-week course of twice-weekly acupuncture and a Chinese herbal formula taken 3 times daily. Primary end points were changes in the Eczema Area and Severity Index, Dermatology Life Quality Index, and patient assessment of itch measured on a visual analog scale. At the end of treatment, all patients had an improvement in AD severity when compared with the baseline. However, whether this score reduction was clinically relevant is uncertain. More than 75% of patients experienced a reduction in pruritus and improvement of quality of life. No adverse effects were observed.

Hochu-ekki-to is a traditional Japanese Kampo medicine which originated in China and is composed of 10 species of medicinal plants. In the framework of Kampo medicine, individuals are categorized as having a particular physiologic constitution. The premise of the study of Hochu-ekki-to for AD is that it has been considered effective for individuals with a Kikyo constitution, which includes atopics. This herbal medicine has been studied in conditions of chronic fatigue (murine model) and chronic obstructive pulmonary disease, as well as in individuals undergoing chemotherapy. In vitro and in vivo studies of this herbal medicine have demonstrated some immunomodulatory properties, such as enhancing mucosal IgA production and attenuating proallergic cytokine IL-4 production.[63]

In a placebo-controlled study, 91 individuals with AD and a Kikyo constitution underwent 24 weeks of intervention (herbal therapy or placebo).[64] All patients continued their regular treatments (topical steroids, topical tacrolimus, emollients, or oral antihistamines) during the study. Hochu-ekki-to or placebo was orally administered twice daily for 24 weeks. Seventy-seven of the initial group completed the trial. Only mild adverse events such as nausea and diarrhea were noted in both groups, without statistical difference. Outcomes included AD severity scores, efficacy, and exacerbation rates. There was no significant reduction in AD severity at the end of the trial. However, there were some promising trends. Although the rate of efficacy did not reach statistical significance ($P = .06$), it was higher in the Hochu-ekki-to group compared with placebo (19% vs 5%). Furthermore, the rate of exacerbation was significantly ($P<.05$) lower in the Hochu-ekki-to group (3%) than in the placebo group (18%). Because the use of topical steroids and tacrolimus was significantly lower at the end of 24 weeks of intervention in the Hochu-ekki-to group, the investigators concluded that this could be a useful adjunct to conventional treatments for patients with AD who have a Kikyo constitution.[64]

Animal Model Studies

A Chinese herbal formula called Bakumijiogan (BJG) has been investigated in an NC/Jic mouse model of AD.[65] AD symptoms were induced by repeated injections of

Dermatophagoides farinae (Df) antigen into the ear auricle for 16 days. Daily oral administration of BJG from 7 days before to 16 days after the first injection significantly reduced ear swelling. BJG was also observed to suppress the total levels of IgE and Df-antigen-specific IgG1 at 17 days after first injection. Serum levels of the T_H1 cytokine IFN-γ and lesional IFN-γ mRNA levels were significantly higher, whereas lesional IL-1α and TNF-α mRNA levels were lower in BJG-treated mice than in control mice.[65]

A Korean herbal medicine called DA-9102 is currently in phase II of clinical investigation. Published data on this medicine are from a murine model (magnesium deficiency–induced AD in hairless rats). Oral administration of DA-9102 at a dose of 100 mg/kg for 16 days was observed to suppress the occurrence of spontaneous dermatitis.[66] Eczematous skin lesions, water loss, and scratching behavior were significantly decreased by DA-9102 in a dose-dependent manner. Results from flow cytometry analysis of PBMCs indicated that DA-9102 suppressed leukocyte activation. DA-9102 not only suppressed the mRNA expression of T_H2 cytokines including IL-4 and IL-10 in the lymph node but also decreased the levels of inflammatory mediators such as nitric oxide and leukotriene B_4 in the serum.[66]

Homeopathy has recently increased in popularity among patients with skin disease. Unlike the traditional herbal medicines discussed under this section of whole medical systems, outcomes for homeopathy are difficult to quantify because the treatments are individualized. A meta-analysis of 89 placebo-controlled trials of homeopathic medicine concluded that the clinical effects of homeopathy in a variety of medical conditions were not placebo effects.[67] Despite this, the researchers surmised that insufficient evidence existed to show that any one type of homeopathic remedy was specifically effective in any clinical condition. A study of individualized homeopathic treatments focused on patients' own assessments of 7 elements (overall impression, improvement of skin condition, reduction of itchiness, reduction of sleep disturbance, satisfaction in daily life, fulfillment at work, and satisfaction in human relations) using a 9-point scale similar to the Glasgow Homeopathic Hospital Outcome Scale.[68] Of the 60 patients, 25 with chronic skin disease had AD. Another 20 had a nonspecific eczema other than AD. Treatment periods ranged between 3 and 31 months. About 50% of individuals with AD reported greater satisfaction in daily life, greater fulfillment at work, and greater satisfaction in human relations.[68]

MIND-BODY
Manipulative and Body-Based Practices

As suggested by observations with homeopathy, there is an inextricable tie between chronic skin conditions and psychological/psychosomatic symptoms. A parasympathetic tone-skewed autonomic balance has been described in atopic diseases, but there are studies refuting this notion.[69] A recent case-control study sought to reevaluate the autonomics in 30 adults with AD.[70] Findings included decreased resting autonomic "set point" (assessed by heart rate variability during 5 minutes at rest) and increased parasympathetic tone in patients with AD when compared with normal controls. Furthermore, individuals with AD had higher values for parasympathetic modulation than healthy controls in response to deep breathing but not in response to postural changes. The investigators interpreted these findings to be consistent with the concept of an altered autonomic set point, while similar tone in the setting of postural change indicated that autonomic function to defined tasks remained intact.[70] Whether these alterations are disease inherent or counterregulatory remains uncertain. Furthermore, there are 2 factors to take into account before attempting to interpret this potential autonomic dysregulation observed in AD. One is the impressive complexity of the efferent signaling pathways of the parasympathetic system.[71] For instance, although the physiologic cholinergic pathway has been described as overall antiinflammatory,[72] increased cholinergic tone does not necessarily equate with purely antiinflammatory effects, as acetylcholine has been shown to promote histamine release from mast cells.[73] Secondly, one cannot discount the influence and interplay of associated psychiatric symptoms/conditions, such as depression and anxiety, which are often associated with decreased vagal tone. The limited volume of literature in this area includes a study of 12 patients with AD who were exposed to a fixed sequence of treatment phases (no treatment, nonspecific treatment factors, electromyographic feedback and relaxation). Significant remission of disease was noted but could not be attributed to a specific phase in the above-mentioned sequence.[74] From the perspective of safety, this area of CAM is less concerning.

SUMMARY

The burden of atopic diseases, including AD, is significant and far-reaching. In addition to cost of care and therapies, it affects the quality of life for those affected as well as their caretakers. Complementary and alternative therapies are commonly used because of concerns about potential adverse effects of conventional therapies and frustration with the lack of response to prescribed medications, be it due to the severity of the AD or the lack of appropriate regular use. Despite the promising results reported with various herbal medicines and biologic products, the clinical efficacy of such alternative therapies remains to be determined. Physicians need to be educated about alternative therapies and discuss benefits and potential adverse effects or limitations with patients. A systematic approach and awareness of reputable and easily accessible resources are helpful in dealing with CAM.

REFERENCES

1. Eisenberg DM. Advising patients who seek alternative medical therapies. Ann Intern Med 1997;127(1):61–9.
2. McNamara SH. FDA regulation of ingredients in dietary supplements after passage of the Dietary Supplement Health and Education Act of 1994: an update. Food Drug Law J 1996;51(2):313–8.
3. Bielory L. Complementary and alternative interventions in asthma, allergy, and immunology. Ann Allergy Asthma Immunol 2004;93(2 Suppl 1):S45–54.
4. Mainardi T, Kapoor S, Bielory L. Complementary and alternative medicine: herbs, phytochemicals and vitamins and their immunologic effects. J Allergy Clin Immunol 2009;123(2):283–94 [quiz 295–86].
5. Bielory L, Lupoli K. Herbal interventions in asthma and allergy. J Asthma 1999; 36(1):1–65.
6. Jensen P. Alternative therapy for atopic dermatitis and psoriasis: patient-reported motivation, information source and effect. Acta Derm Venereol 1990;70(5):425–8.
7. Hughes R, Ward D, Tobin AM, et al. The use of alternative medicine in pediatric patients with atopic dermatitis. Pediatr Dermatol 2007;24(2):118–20.
8. Anderson PC, Dinulos JG. Atopic dermatitis and alternative management strategies. Curr Opin Pediatr 2009;21(1):131–8.
9. Kang KD, Kang SM, Yim HB. Herbal medication aggravates cataract formation: a case report. J Korean Med Sci 2008;23(3):537–9.
10. Ferguson JE, Chalmers RJ, Rowlands DJ. Reversible dilated cardiomyopathy following treatment of atopic eczema with Chinese herbal medicine. Br J Dermatol 1997;136(4):592–3.

11. Ernst E. Adverse effects of herbal drugs in dermatology. Br J Dermatol 2000; 143(5):923–9.
12. Engler RJ, With CM, Gregory PJ, et al. Complementary and alternative medicine for the allergist-immunologist: where do I start? J Allergy Clin Immunol 2009; 123(2):309–16.
13. Ramsay HM, Goddard W, Gill S, et al. Herbal creams used for atopic eczema in Birmingham, UK illegally contain potent corticosteroids. Arch Dis Child 2003; 88(12):1056–7.
14. Smits HH, Engering A, van der Kleij D, et al. Selective probiotic bacteria induce IL-10-producing regulatory T cells in vitro by modulating dendritic cell function through dendritic cell-specific intercellular adhesion molecule 3-grabbing nonintegrin. J Allergy Clin Immunol 2005;115(6):1260–7.
15. Prescott SL, Dunstan JA, Hale J, et al. Clinical effects of probiotics are associated with increased interferon-gamma responses in very young children with atopic dermatitis. Clin Exp Allergy 2005;35(12):1557–64.
16. Rautava S, Kalliomaki M, Isolauri E. New therapeutic strategy for combating the increasing burden of allergic disease: Probiotics-A Nutrition, Allergy, Mucosal Immunology and Intestinal Microbiota (NAMI) Research Group report. J Allergy Clin Immunol 2005;116(1):31–7.
17. Kalliomaki M, Salminen S, Arvilommi H, et al. Probiotics in primary prevention of atopic disease: a randomised placebo-controlled trial. Lancet 2001;357(9262): 1076–9.
18. Kalliomaki M, Salminen S, Poussa T, et al. Probiotics and prevention of atopic disease: 4-year follow-up of a randomised placebo-controlled trial. Lancet 2003;361(9372):1869–71.
19. Kopp MV, Hennemuth I, Heinzmann A, et al. Randomized, double-blind, placebo-controlled trial of probiotics for primary prevention: no clinical effects of Lactobacillus GG supplementation. Pediatrics 2008;121(4):e850–6.
20. Taylor AL, Dunstan JA, Prescott SL. Probiotic supplementation for the first 6 months of life fails to reduce the risk of atopic dermatitis and increases the risk of allergen sensitization in high-risk children: a randomized controlled trial. J Allergy Clin Immunol 2007;119(1):184–91.
21. Soh SE, Aw M, Gerez I, et al. Probiotic supplementation in the first 6 months of life in at risk Asian infants–effects on eczema and atopic sensitization at the age of 1 year. Clin Exp Allergy 2009;39(4):571–8.
22. Tang ML. Probiotics and prebiotics: immunological and clinical effects in allergic disease. Nestle Nutr Workshop Ser Pediatr Program 2009;64:219–38.
23. van der Aa LB, Heymans HS, van Aalderen WM, et al. Probiotics and prebiotics in atopic dermatitis: review of the theoretical background and clinical evidence. Pediatr Allergy Immunol 2009;21(2):e355–67.
24. Kopp MV, Salfeld P. Probiotics and prevention of allergic disease. Curr Opin Clin Nutr Metab Care 2009;12(3):298–303.
25. Kuitunen M, Kukkonen K, Juntunen-Backman K, et al. Probiotics prevent IgE-associated allergy until age 5 years in cesarean-delivered children but not in the total cohort. J Allergy Clin Immunol 2009;123(2):335–41.
26. Kukkonen K, Savilahti E, Haahtela T, et al. Probiotics and prebiotic galacto-oligosaccharides in the prevention of allergic diseases: a randomized, double-blind, placebo-controlled trial. J Allergy Clin Immunol 2007;119(1):192–8.
27. Moro G, Arslanoglu S, Stahl B, et al. A mixture of prebiotic oligosaccharides reduces the incidence of atopic dermatitis during the first six months of age. Arch Dis Child 2006;91(10):814–9.

28. Ziegler E, Vanderhoof JA, Petschow B, et al. Term infants fed formula supplemented with selected blends of prebiotics grow normally and have soft stools similar to those reported for breast-fed infants. J Pediatr Gastroenterol Nutr 2007;44(3):359–64.

29. Weston S, Halbert A, Richmond P, et al. Effects of probiotics on atopic dermatitis: a randomised controlled trial. Arch Dis Child 2005;90(9):892–7.

30. Volz T, Biedermann T. [Outside-in: probiotic topical agents]. Hautarzt 2009; 60(10):795–801 [in German].

31. Rowe A, Farrell AM, Bunker CB. Constitutive endothelial and inducible nitric oxide synthase in inflammatory dermatoses. Br J Dermatol 1997;136(1):18–23.

32. Taniuchi S, Kojima T, Hara Mt K, et al. Increased serum nitrate levels in infants with atopic dermatitis. Allergy 2001;56(7):693–5.

33. Morita H, Semma M, Hori M, et al. Clinical application of nitric oxide synthase inhibitor for atopic dermatitis. Int J Dermatol 1995;34(4):294–5.

34. Stucker M, Pieck C, Stoerb C, et al. Topical vitamin B12–a new therapeutic approach in atopic dermatitis-evaluation of efficacy and tolerability in a randomized placebo-controlled multicentre clinical trial. Br J Dermatol 2004;150(5):977–83.

35. Erkkola M, Kaila M, Nwaru BI, et al. Maternal vitamin D intake during pregnancy is inversely associated with asthma and allergic rhinitis in 5-year-old children. Clin Exp Allergy 2009;39(6):875–82.

36. Back O, Blomquist HK, Hernell O, et al. Does vitamin D intake during infancy promote the development of atopic allergy? Acta Derm Venereol 2009;89(1): 28–32.

37. Patrizi A, Raone B, Neri I. Atopiclair. Expert Opin Pharmacother 2009;10(7): 1223–30.

38. Patrizi A, Capitanio B, Neri I, et al. A double-blind, randomized, vehicle-controlled clinical study to evaluate the efficacy and safety of MAS063DP (ATOPICLAIR) in the management of atopic dermatitis in paediatric patients. Pediatr Allergy Immunol 2008;19(7):619–25.

39. Niwa Y, Tominaga K, Yoshida K. Successful treatment of severe atopic dermatitis-complicated cataract and male infertility with a natural product antioxidant. Int J Tissue React 1998;20(2):63–9.

40. Lovell CR, Burton JL, Horrobin DF. Treatment of atopic eczema with evening primrose oil. Lancet 1981;1(8214):278.

41. Wright S, Burton JL. Oral evening-primrose-seed oil improves atopic eczema. Lancet 1982;2(8308):1120–2.

42. Bamford JT, Gibson RW, Renier CM. Atopic eczema unresponsive to evening primrose oil (linoleic and gamma-linolenic acids). J Am Acad Dermatol 1985; 13(6):959–65.

43. Henz BM, Jablonska S, van de Kerkhof PC, et al. Double-blind, multicentre analysis of the efficacy of borage oil in patients with atopic eczema. Br J Dermatol 1999;140(4):685–8.

44. Skogh M. Atopic eczema unresponsive to evening primrose oil (linoleic and gamma-linolenic acids). J Am Acad Dermatol 1986;15(1):114–5.

45. Biagi PL, Bordoni A, Masi M, et al. A long-term study on the use of evening primrose oil (Efamol) in atopic children. Drugs Exp Clin Res 1988;14(4):285–90.

46. Schalin-Karrila M, Mattila L, Jansen CT, et al. Evening primrose oil in the treatment of atopic eczema: effect on clinical status, plasma phospholipid fatty acids and circulating blood prostaglandins. Br J Dermatol 1987;117(1):11–9.

47. Stonemetz D. A review of the clinical efficacy of evening primrose. Holist Nurs Pract 2008;22(3):171–4.

48. Takwale A, Tan E, Agarwal S, et al. Efficacy and tolerability of borage oil in adults and children with atopic eczema: randomised, double blind, placebo controlled, parallel group trial. BMJ 2003;327(7428):1385.
49. van Gool CJ, Thijs C, Henquet CJ, et al. Gamma-linolenic acid supplementation for prophylaxis of atopic dermatitis–a randomized controlled trial in infants at high familial risk. Am J Clin Nutr 2003;77(4):943–51.
50. Schempp CM, Windeck T, Hezel S, et al. Topical treatment of atopic dermatitis with St. John's wort cream–a randomized, placebo controlled, double blind half-side comparison. Phytomedicine 2003;10(Suppl 4):31–7.
51. Kotani M, Matsumoto M, Fujita A, et al. Persimmon leaf extract and astragalin inhibit development of dermatitis and IgE elevation in NC/Nga mice. J Allergy Clin Immunol 2000;106(1 Pt 1):159–66.
52. Matsumoto M, Kotani M, Fujita A, et al. Oral administration of persimmon leaf extract ameliorates skin symptoms and transepidermal water loss in atopic dermatitis model mice, NC/Nga. Br J Dermatol 2002;146(2):221–7.
53. Qi XF, Kim DH, Yoon YS, et al. Effects of Bambusae caulis in Liquamen on the development of atopic dermatitis-like skin lesions in hairless mice. J Ethnopharmacol 2009;123(2):195–200.
54. Joo SS, Won TJ, Nam SY, et al. Therapeutic advantages of medicinal herbs fermented with Lactobacillus plantarum, in topical application and its activities on atopic dermatitis. Phytother Res 2009;23(7):913–9.
55. Fung AY, Look PC, Chong LY, et al. A controlled trial of traditional Chinese herbal medicine in Chinese patients with recalcitrant atopic dermatitis. Int J Dermatol 1999;38(5):387–92.
56. Zhang W, Leonard T, Bath-Hextall F, et al. Chinese herbal medicine for atopic eczema. Cochrane Database Syst Rev 2005;(2):CD002291.
57. Hon KL, Leung TF, Wong Y, et al. A pentaherbs capsule as a treatment option for atopic dermatitis in children: an open-labeled case series. Am J Chin Med 2004; 32(6):941–50.
58. Hon KL, Lee VW, Leung TF, et al. Corticosteroids are not present in a traditional Chinese medicine formulation for atopic dermatitis in children. Ann Acad Med Singapore 2006;35(11):759–63.
59. Hon KL, Leung TF, Ng PC, et al. Efficacy and tolerability of a Chinese herbal medicine concoction for treatment of atopic dermatitis: a randomized, double-blind, placebo-controlled study. Br J Dermatol 2007;157(2):357–63.
60. Leung TF, Wong KY, Wong CK, et al. In vitro and clinical immunomodulatory effects of a novel Pentaherbs concoction for atopic dermatitis. Br J Dermatol 2008;158(6):1216–23.
61. Chan BC, Hon KL, Leung PC, et al. Traditional Chinese medicine for atopic eczema: PentaHerbs formula suppresses inflammatory mediators release from mast cells. J Ethnopharmacol 2008;120(1):85–91.
62. Salameh F, Perla D, Solomon M, et al. The effectiveness of combined Chinese herbal medicine and acupuncture in the treatment of atopic dermatitis. J Altern Complement Med 2008;14(8):1043–8.
63. Nakada T, Watanabe K, Matsumoto T, et al. Effect of orally administered Hochu-ekki-to, a Japanese herbal medicine, on contact hypersensitivity caused by repeated application of antigen. Int Immunopharmacol 2002;2(7): 901–11.
64. Kobayashi H, Ishii M, Takeuchi S, et al. Efficacy and safety of a traditional herbal medicine, Hochu-ekki-to in the long-term management of Kikyo (delicate constitution) patients with atopic dermatitis: a 6-month, multicenter, double-blind,

randomized, placebo-controlled study. Evid Based Complement Alternat Med 2008. [Epub ahead of print].

65. Makino T, Hamanaka M, Yamashita H, et al. Effect of bakumijiogan, an herbal formula in traditional Chinese medicine, on atopic dermatitis-like skin lesions induced by mite antigen in NC/Jic mice. Biol Pharm Bull 2008;31(11):2108–13.

66. Choi JJ, Park B, Kim DH, et al. Blockade of atopic dermatitis-like skin lesions by DA-9102, a natural medicine isolated from Actinidia arguta, in the Mg-deficiency induced dermatitis model of hairless rats. Exp Biol Med (Maywood) 2008;233(8): 1026–34.

67. Linde K, Clausius N, Ramirez G, et al. Are the clinical effects of homeopathy placebo effects? A meta-analysis of placebo-controlled trials. Lancet 1997; 350(9081):834–43.

68. Itamura R. Effect of homeopathic treatment of 60 Japanese patients with chronic skin disease. Complement Ther Med 2007;15(2):115–20.

69. Murphy GM, Smith SE, Smith SA, et al. Autonomic function in cholinergic urticaria and atopic eczema. Br J Dermatol 1984;110(5):581–6.

70. Boettger MK, Bar KJ, Dohrmann A, et al. Increased vagal modulation in atopic dermatitis. J Dermatol Sci 2009;53(1):55–9.

71. Tracey KJ. Physiology and immunology of the cholinergic antiinflammatory pathway. J Clin Invest 2007;117(2):289–96.

72. Wang H, Yu M, Ochani M, et al. Nicotinic acetylcholine receptor alpha7 subunit is an essential regulator of inflammation. Nature 2003;421(6921):384–8.

73. Masini E, Fantozzi R, Conti A, et al. Immunological modulation of cholinergic histamine release in isolated rat mast cells. Agents Actions 1985;16(3–4):152–4.

74. Haynes SN, Wilson CC, Jaffe PG, et al. Biofeedback treatment of atopic dermatitis: controlled case studies of eight cases. Biofeedback Self Regul 1979;4(3): 195–209.

Investigational and Unproven Therapies in Atopic Dermatitis

Peck Y. Ong, MD[a,b],*, Mark Boguniewicz, MD[c]

KEYWORDS

• Atopic dermatitis • Treatment • Experimental therapy

Atopic dermatitis (AD) is a common chronic inflammatory skin disease that affects up to 20% of children and 2% of adults worldwide in both developed and developing countries.[1] The significant effect of the disease on patients and their caregivers has been well documented[2,3] (see also the article by Chamlin and Chren elsewhere in this issue for further exploration of this topic), as has the economic effect on families and society.[4,5] Although patients with milder disease may respond to several conventional therapies, new therapeutic interventions are needed for those patients in whom the disease is difficult to control.

CONVENTIONAL THERAPY

AD is a complex disease with multifactorial causes, including skin barrier defects and immune dysregulation with irritant, allergic, and infectious triggers.[6–8] Avoidance of proven triggers (see the article by Caubet and Eigenmann elsewhere in this issue for further exploration of this topic), along with proper skin hydration and moisturization, forms the foundation of conventional therapy.[9] Topical corticosteroids (TCSs) remain the first-line anti-inflammatory therapy for symptomatic treatment of AD.[10] However, nonadherence in using TCSs remains an important barrier in the treatment of AD, with patients or caregivers often delaying use of the TCSs for up to 7 days after onset of flare.[11–13] Nonsteroidal medications include the topical calcineurin inhibitors (TCIs) pimecrolimus cream 1% (Elidel) and tacrolimus ointment 0.03% and 0.1% (Protopic). These medications are currently indicated as second-line treatment for intermittent, noncontinuous use in children aged 2 years and older with moderate to severe AD (tacrolimus ointment 0.03%) and mild to moderate AD (pimecrolimus cream 1%).

[a] Division of Clinical Immunology and Allergy, Childrens Hospital Los Angeles, 4650, Sunset Boulevard, MS #75, Los Angeles, CA 90027, USA
[b] Department of Pediatrics, Keck School of Medicine, University of Southern California, Los Angeles, CA, USA
[c] Division of Allergy-Immunology, Department of Pediatrics, National Jewish Health and University of Colorado School of Medicine, 1400, Jackson Street, Denver, CO 80206, USA
* Corresponding author. 4650, Childrens Hospital Los Angeles, MS# 75, Los Angeles, CA 90027.
E-mail address: pyong@chla.usc.edu

Immunol Allergy Clin N Am 30 (2010) 425–439
doi:10.1016/j.iac.2010.05.002
0889-8561/10/$ – see front matter © 2010 Elsevier Inc. All rights reserved.

Tacrolimus ointment 0.1% is indicated for patients 16 years and older. Despite well-documented safety,[14–16] their use significantly decreased after a boxed warning issued by the Food and Drug Administration (FDA) that long-term use may be associated with risk of cancer. Evolution in conventional therapy using a proactive approach with both TCSs and TCIs is reviewed by Wollenberg and Schnopp elsewhere in this issue. Newer nonsteroidal creams registered as medical devices, thus requiring a prescription despite not being FDA-regulated, include Atopiclair, Eletone, EpiCeram, and MimyX.[17] These creams have no age or length-of-use restrictions; however, they are expensive, and comparison with topical treatments has been limited.[18]

For patients with severe AD, systemic immunosuppressive drugs, including cyclosporine, mycophenolate mofetil, azathioprine, and methotrexate, have been shown to be effective, although serious adverse events limit their use, especially in pediatric patients.[10,19] Other approaches include ultraviolet (UV) phototherapy[20] and wet-wrap therapy.[21] The latter may be especially effective when incorporated into a comprehensive management program.[22] An important clinical point is that successful outcomes in the management of patients with AD are strongly tied to proper education of patients and caregivers (see the article by Nicol and Ersser elsewhere in this issue for further exploration of this topic).

INVESTIGATIONAL OR UNPROVEN THERAPIES
Barrier Therapy

The goal of barrier therapy in AD is to repair an abnormal epidermal barrier and prevent barrier dysfunction.[23] Loss-of-function mutations in the filaggrin gene have been shown to be associated with reduced levels of natural moisturizing factor in the stratum corneum.[24] In a recent randomized, controlled, prospective study, Wirén and colleagues[25] showed that a barrier-strengthening cream containing urea (Canoderm cream 5%) was capable of delaying the relapse of AD in patients who had been treated with TCSs. The subjects were first treated with betamethasone valerate cream 0.1% on defined areas of eczema for 3 weeks; they were then randomized to receive Canoderm or no treatment. Over a 6-month period, 68% of the treated group had no relapse of eczema versus 32% of the untreated group (P<.01). However, skin barrier function, as measured by transepidermal water loss (TEWL), was not significantly different between the 2 groups. The study highlights the importance of barrier treatment in the prevention of symptoms in established AD. However, larger studies and comparison with other barrier treatments are needed to confirm these results.

A study of extracts prepared from silica mud and 2 different microalgae species derived from a specific geothermal biotope in Iceland known to be beneficial for patients with AD showed them to be capable of inducing filaggrin and other epidermal barrier gene expression in primary human epidermal keratinocytes.[26] In addition, a formulation containing all 3 extracts induced identical gene regulatory effects in vivo, associated with a significant reduction of TEWL when applied topically to normal skin in healthy subjects.

Antistaphylococcal Treatments

Because Staphylococcus aureus appears to play an important role in the pathogenesis of AD inflammation,[8] strategies to decrease colonization and neutralize effects of superantigenic toxins with superantigenic properties would be especially important. The emergence of methicillin-resistant S aureus (MRSA) as an increasingly common pathogen in patients with AD underscores the urgency of developing new treatments in this area.[27]

Antimicrobial fabrics

Silver- or antimicrobial-coated fabrics have been found to be effective in the treatment of AD.[17] More recently, in an explorative 8-week study, Fluhr and colleagues[28] showed that silver-loaded seaweed fiber clothing significantly decreased *S aureus* colonization in patients with AD compared with cotton garments. In addition, the group with silver-loaded seaweed fiber clothing had significant improvement in their skin barrier function in areas of mild eczema during the initial 4 weeks of treatment as compared with the cotton fiber group. The investigators hypothesized that an antioxidative effect of the silver-loaded seaweed fiber contributed to clinical benefit. Of note, they showed that there was no deleterious effect of the active treatment on commensal bacteria. This observation may be of clinical importance, given recent data that showed that *Staphylococcus epidermidis* may play a beneficial anti-inflammatory role in cutaneous inflammation.[29] Further studies are needed to compare the clinical improvement of AD and potential side effects using these fabrics.

Bleach baths

Huang and colleagues[30] confirmed the efficacy of bleach bath in AD in a randomized, investigator-blinded, placebo-controlled study. In this pediatric study, 15 children with AD were randomized to treatment with diluted bleach (0.005%) twice weekly along with nasal mupirocin added for 5 days each month versus 16 patients with AD treated with water twice weekly and application of nasal petrolatum. After 3 months, AD severity based on the eczema area and severity index (EASI), body surface area involved, and Investigator's Global Assessment improved significantly in the bleach bath–treated group. Of note, there was no significant difference in the AD severity on body parts (head and neck) that were not submerged in the bleach bath. There were no significant adverse events noted, and no patients withdrew from the study because of their intolerance to the baths. This treatment might be especially useful for patients with recurrent MRSA infections. Unfortunately, this study did not address this question and, in addition, patients on active treatment remained colonized by *S aureus*. It is worth noting that many patients with AD, especially those with open and inflamed lesions, do not tolerate even dilute bleach baths.

Topical antiseptics

Topical antiseptics remain an attractive antistaphylococcal treatment for AD because of their low risk of causing bacterial resistance. However, a well-known side effect of antiseptics is their potential for causing local irritation or sensitivity. In a double-blind randomized study, Wohlrab and colleagues[31] used a combination of 2 topical antiseptics, triclosan 0.3% and chlorhexidine 0.34%, in lower concentrations in a carrier emulsion for topical treatment of AD and compared it to topical triclosan 2% in the same carrier emulsion. These investigators found that the low-concentration combination therapy led to a similar reduction in AD severity as the higher-concentration single antiseptic at a 2-week follow-up, with a similar reduction in bacterial counts. However, comparison of adverse events was not reported.

In a more recent randomized, double-blind controlled trial, Tan and colleagues[32] showed that an emollient containing 1% triclosan had TCS-sparing effects in patients with mild to moderate AD compared with the emollient alone. Patients applied either the emollient alone or emollient with 1% triclosan on the whole body twice daily for 27 days. Both groups were allowed to apply betamethasone valerate cream 0.025% on the affected areas. The investigators had a follow-up on days 14, 27, and 41. AD severity measured by the scoring atopic dermatitis (SCORAD) index significantly improved on day 14 in the group using triclosan compared with the group using only emollient. AD severity continued to improve in both groups, and there was no significant difference in AD severity between them on days 27 and 41. However, there was significantly less use of TCSs in the group taking triclosan than in the group taking only emollient over the 41-day study period ($P<.05$). Three subjects in the triclosan group experienced local stinging pain after application of the topical preparation compared with none in the emollient group. The stinging pain, however, resolved with continued use of the cream, and no subject withdrew from the study as a result of any an adverse effects.

Specific antibodies and vaccines

Community acquired (CA)-MRSA infections have become increasingly common among patients with AD.[27] An important virulence regulator in staphylococci that characterizes CA-MRSA strains is the accessory gene regulator agr.[33] Agr signals through an exported autoinducing peptide (AIP), and antibodies designed against the AIP of one S aureus agr subgroup have been shown to specifically prevent agr expression and S aureus disease in an animal model of abscess formation.[34] Of note, these antibodies also provided protection when administered before infection.

Devising new therapeutic strategies to combat S aureus is complicated by the infection not being associated with the development of protective immunity to any significant degree, partly because our immune system has ongoing exposure to staphylococcal antigens and many strains are commensal organisms. In addition, S aureus produces protein A to help it evade acquired host defense. Although several attempts to develop protective vaccines have met with failure in clinical trials, a new conjugated vaccine (PentaStaph) that includes α-toxin and Panton-Valentine leukocidin is currently in clinical trials. In addition, positive results based on using a combination of systematically selected antigens have been reported.[35] These combinatory vaccines target microbial surface components recognizing adhesive matrix molecules (MSCRAMMs), a family of bacterial proteins that bind to human extracellular matrix components. Stranger-Jones and colleagues[36] developed a vaccine based on a combination of antigens that provided complete protection from lethal doses of S aureus in a murine challenge model. Of importance, MSCRAMM vaccines have been shown to prevent colonization.[37] Their clinical benefit in patients with AD remains to be determined.

Another promising antigenic target for vaccine development against S aureus is teichoic acid, which has been implicated in nasal colonization and biofilm formation.[38] In a recent study of children with impetiginized AD, significant levels of lipoteichoic acid were measured in infected lesions, which were able to induce epidermal cytokine gene expression ex vivo.[39]

Antistaphylococcal toxin strategies

Ultimately, treatment may need to be directed at eliminating or neutralizing exotoxins secreted by S aureus that contribute to the chronic inflammation and severity of AD.[7] Initial attempts at neutralizing staphylococcal enterotoxin B (SEB) with soluble high-affinity receptor antagonists appear to be promising.[40] Of importance, this group was also able to express Vβ domains in tandem as a single-chain protein demonstrating the feasibility of engineering a broader spectrum antagonist capable of neutralizing multiple toxins, including the clinically important superantigens, SEB and toxic shock syndrome toxin 1.[41]

Ceragenins

Besides problems with S aureus, patients with AD, even those with quiescent disease, have a unique susceptibility to eczema vaccinatum.[42] This potentially lethal reaction to immunization with smallpox vaccine (vaccinia virus [VV]) may be related to a deficiency of antimicrobial peptides (AMPs).[43] Although cathelicidins and human β-defensin 3 exhibit potent antiviral activity against VV,[44] their use as anti-VV agents is limited because of rapid degradation by endogenous tissue proteases. Ceragenins are synthetic antimicrobial compounds designed to mimic the structure and function of endogenous AMPs.[45] Ceragenins have been shown to disrupt bacterial membranes without damaging mammalian cell membranes.[46] As a result of their synthetic nature, ceragenins are not subject to human protease degradation and therefore have a longer tissue half-life. One ceragenin compound (cationic steroid antimicrobial [CSA] 13) was recently shown to exhibit potent antiviral activity against VV via direct antiviral effects and by stimulating the expression of endogenous AMPs with known antiviral activity.[47] In addition, topical application of CSA-13 resulted in reduced satellite lesion formation, suggesting the use of CSA-13 as an acute intervention for patients with disseminated VV skin infection.

Anti-Inflammatory Therapies and Immunomodulation

Chemokine antagonists

An important role for chemokines in the pathogenesis of AD has emerged.[48] Increased levels of CCL17 and CCL22 have consistently been shown to correlate with increased severity or disease activity of AD.[49] Both CCL17 and CCL22 bind to CCR4 receptor to exert their chemotactic effects on leukocytes, and blocking CCR4 presents an opportunity to antagonize the action of these 2 chemokines. Nakagami and colleagues[50] showed that the novel compound RS-1154 competed with CCL17 in binding to human CCR4. In a mouse model, the investigators demonstrated that orally administered RS-1154 was capable of inhibiting ovalbumin-induced ear swelling caused by CCL17 and CCL22. CCR3 is another chemokine receptor that mediates allergic inflammation.[51] Suzuki and colleagues[52] found that the CCR3 antagonist YM-344031 significantly decreased ovalbumin-induced murine ear edema compared with vehicle. The anti-inflammatory effect of YM-344031 was similar to that of prednisolone. Taken together, these animal studies illustrate the potential value of chemokine antagonists for future human trials in the treatment of AD.

Transcription factor decoy oligodeoxynucleotides

Transcription factors are essential intracellular molecules in the inflammatory pathways. In murine models of AD, a topical decoy oligodeoxynucleotide (ODN) has been used to block NF-κB, a key transcription factor in inflammation.[17] More recently, Igawa and colleagues[53] conducted an open-label pilot study using topical decoy ODN ointment to block STAT6, a transcription factor critical in allergic inflammation, in 10 adult patients with moderate to severe AD. Each subject applied the topical STAT6 decoy ODN ointment to one side, with paired lesions treated with a control emollient. Both the EASI scores and visual analog scale (VAS), a measure of pruritus, decreased significantly on the side receiving active treatment at the 2- and 4-week visits ($P<.05$).

Interleukin-4 and interleukin-13 antagonists

Interleukin (IL)-4 and IL-13 are T-cell–derived cytokines that play an important role in acute AD.[7] Aeroderm, an IL-4 mutein, interferes with the IL-4α receptor, blocking both IL-4 and IL-13. In a randomized, double-blind, placebo-controlled trial of adult patients with moderate to severe AD, the drug was given twice daily for 28 days by subcutaneous injection.[54] Although the group treated with Aeroderm showed greater reduction in disease severity versus the placebo group, this was not a statistically significant difference. However, the active treatment group did have statistically significant decrease in eczema exacerbations. More recently, Morioka and colleagues[55] studied the effect of murine IL-4 double mutant (DM), an IL-4 antagonist DNA capable of inhibiting the activity of IL-4 and IL-13. IL-4DM significantly suppressed oxazolone-induced ear swelling and dermatitis in the mouse model of AD compared with the control DNA-treated group. The group treated with IL-4DM also had significantly lower plasma IgE and histamine than the control group.

Suplatast tosilate
Suplatast tosilate is a Th2 cytokine inhibitor. Systemic administration of suplatast tosilate has been shown to be beneficial in AD.[56] In addition, topical therapy with suplatast tosilate ointment 3% inhibits the expression of IL-4 and IL-5 and ameliorates skin manifestations in a murine model of AD, suggesting potential usefulness for the treatment of AD.[57] A meta-analysis showed that suplatast/tacrolimus combination therapy resulted in better improvement in skin symptom scores and significantly decreased the dose of tacrolimus compared with topical tacrolimus alone.[58] In addition, a significantly greater number of patients were able to discontinue tacrolimus ointment by using the combination therapy with suplatast tosilate versus tacrolimus monotherapy for refractory facial erythema.

Peroxisome proliferator–activated receptor agonists
Peroxisome proliferator–activated receptors (PPARs) are nuclear hormone receptors that are expressed in a variety of cells, including keratinocytes and cells of the immune system that have potential anti-inflammatory activity and function in epidermal repair. In a retrospective review of 6 patients with severe AD, Behshad and colleagues[59] found that orally administered rosiglitazone, a PPAR-γ agonist approved for use in type 2 diabetes mellitus, significantly improved severity of AD when used concomitantly with oral corticosteroid or wet-wrap treatment in some subjects. Rosiglitazone had steroid-sparing effects in patients with severe AD. The dosage used ranged from 2 to 4 mg twice daily for up to 2 years. A significant side effect observed in the study was weight gain, although other potential side effects included edema, cardiovascular risk, and hepatotoxicity. Two more recent studies using PPAR agonists were done in mouse models of AD. The topically applied PPAR-α agonist WY14643 significantly decreased cutaneous inflammation accompanied by decreased infiltration of CD4 cells, mast cells, and eosinophils and decreased levels of the inflammatory cytokines IL-1β, IL-31, IL-4, interferon (IFN)-γ, and CCL11.[60] In another study, Hatano and colleagues[61] showed that topically applied agonists of PPAR-α, PPAR-β/δ, and liver X receptor–α/β significantly reduced epidermal hyperplasia and inflammation. These investigators also found that these agonists led to significant reduction in TEWL, cutaneous infiltration of eosinophils and mast cells, serum CCL17, and systemic Th2 cells. However, they could not confirm the effectiveness of a PPAR-γ agonist in this mouse model. A role for PPAR agonists in AD remains to be fully defined.

RDP58
RDP58 is a novel immunomodulating decapeptide discovered through activity-based screening and computer-aided rational design.[62] It disrupts cellular responses signaled through the toll-like and tumor necrosis factor (TNF) receptor families and occludes important signal transduction pathways involved in inflammation, inhibiting the production of TNF-α, IFN-γ, IL-2, IL-6, and IL-12. These proinflammatory cytokines are thought to be involved in the pathogenesis of several inflammatory and autoimmune diseases, including AD. Topical application of RDP58 to the epidermis resulted in amelioration of phorbol ester–induced irritant dermatitis.[62] Substantial reductions were observed in skin thickness, inflammatory cytokine production, and other histopathological parameters. RDP58 was also effective in reducing the

compounding inflammatory damage brought on by chronic 12-O-tetradecanoylphorbol 13-acetate exposure, and was capable of targeting inflammatory mediators specifically in keratinocytes. These results suggest that topical RDP58 is an effective anti-inflammatory agent with therapeutic potential in immune-mediated cutaneous diseases such as AD.

Intravenous immunoglobulin
High-dose intravenous immunoglobulin (IVIG) has been shown to have immunomodulatory activity in AD and, in addition, IVIG can interact directly with microbes or toxins involved in the pathogenesis of AD. IVIG has been shown to contain high concentrations of staphylococcal toxin-specific antibodies that inhibit the in vitro activation of T cells by staphylococcal toxins.[63] Treatment of severe refractory AD with IVIG has yielded conflicting results. Studies have not been controlled and have involved small numbers of patients.[64] Although children appear to have a better response than adults, controlled studies are needed to answer the question of efficacy in a more definitive manner.

Omalizumab
Anti-inflammatory effects of monoclonal anti-IgE suggest a role for IgE in allergic inflammation.[65] Several case reports suggest there are clinical benefits of using omalizumab (monoclonal anti-IgE) in some patients with AD, including children treated for their asthma.[66] Treatment of adult patients with severe AD and significantly elevated serum IgE levels did not show benefit when omalizumab was used as monotherapy.[67] By contrast, significant improvement in 3 adolescent patients with AD was observed when omalizumab was added to usual therapy.[68] In an open study of 11 adult patients with high IgE levels treated with anti-IgE, some patients had very good clinical improvement, others had none, and several had worsening of AD based on change in SCORAD.[69] Specific markers have not been found to identify potential responders, and at present the use of omalizumab is not indicated for AD.

Allergen-specific immunotherapy
Specific immunotherapy with aeroallergens is currently not indicated for AD. Although there are anecdotal reports of disease improvement, some patients also report exacerbations of eczema. More recently, Werfel and colleagues[70] showed that in adults with long-standing AD sensitized to dust mite allergen, specific immunotherapy with house dust mite allergen over 12 months resulted in clinical improvement and reduction in topical steroid use. In patients with AD having clinical improvement with subcutaneous allergen-specific immunotherapy (SCIT), Bussmann and colleagues[71] showed that levels of the tolerogenic cytokine IL-10 increased, whereas CCL17 and IL-16 decreased in the sera of the patients during SCIT. Allergen-specific IgE decreased whereas IgG4 increased during SCIT. Preliminary studies with sublingual immunotherapy suggest a role for a subset of children with AD sensitized to dust mite allergen.[72] These data need to be reproduced in a larger pediatric population, especially in light of the natural history of AD.

Vitamin D and heliotherapy
Use of topical vitamin D in AD has been controversial. In a mouse model of IgE-mediated cutaneous reactions, Katayama and colleagues[73] showed that a topical vitamin D_3 ointment was capable of inhibiting both immediate- and late-phase hypersensitivity reactions in the mouse model. However, in a different murine model, Li and colleagues[74] showed that topical application of vitamin D_3 or its analogue, calcipotriol (MC903; Dovonex), increased the production of thymic stromal lymphopoietin,

a cytokine associated with Th2 responses and IgE production, and led to the development of eczematous changes. The investigators observed increased pruritus, epidermal hyperplasia, and increased numbers of cutaneous eosinophils and systemic IgE, similar to findings in patients with AD.

The skin is crucial for synthesizing vitamin D after exposure to sunlight. Because people in Scandinavia have limited exposure to sunlight in the winter and are at risk for seasonal vitamin D insufficiency, a group of Finnish researchers hypothesized that heliotherapy may lead to increased vitamin D production and improvement of AD during the winter.[75] Their study included 23 adult patients with AD who received heliotherapy for 2 weeks either in January or March in the Canary Islands. The investigators showed that both groups had significantly increased serum concentration of calcidiol, the circulating form of vitamin D, after heliotherapy. Both groups had significant improvement of AD severity based on a decrease in SCORAD after heliotherapy. In addition, there was a positive correlation in the improvement of serum calcidiol concentration and SCORAD in the group receiving heliotherapy in March. The improvement of AD after heliotherapy shown in this study was consistent with another study[76] and provided indirect support for the beneficial effect of vitamin D in AD. However, benefits need to be weighed against potential long-term adverse effects of heliotherapy, including the development of skin cancer. To improve winter-related AD without exposure to potentially harmful UV radiation, a pilot randomized, double-blind placebo-controlled study was performed with oral supplementation of vitamin D from February to March in Boston, Masachussets.[77] Eleven pediatric patients with mostly mild AD were enrolled. Subjects were assigned to take either vitamin D (1000 international unit [IU] ergocalciferol) or placebo once daily for a month. The Investigator's Global Assessment score improved in 4 of 6 subjects in the group taking vitamin D (80%) compared with 1 of 5 subjects in the group taking placebo ($P = $ .04). There was a larger reduction in EASI score of the vitamin D group compared with the placebo group, but the difference was not statistically significant.

Cutaneous lesions in patients with AD have significantly decreased expression of AMPs compared with psoriatic lesions.[78] This decreased expression may contribute to increased S aureus infections observed in AD compared with psoriasis.[79] In a controlled study, 14 healthy subjects and 14 subjects with AD were supplemented with 4000 IU per day of oral vitamin D_3 (cholecalciferol) for 3 weeks.[80] Expression of the AMP cathelicidin was significantly increased in the skin biopsy specimens of AD lesions compared with those in healthy skin or uninvolved skin in AD. Although the study did not document changes in AD severity or bacterial counts with this treatment, it has implications for a role of oral vitamin D in improving innate immune responses in patients with AD, leading to decreased skin infections and clinical improvement. Sponsored by National Institutes of Health, a multicenter trial of oral vitamin D supplementation is currently being conducted (see the article by Searing and Leung elsewhere in this issue for further exploration of this topic).

Mycobacterium vaccae vaccine
AD is characterized systemically by a predominant Th2 response. Thus, one treatment strategy involves the shifting of a Th2 to a Th1 response. Because mycobacterial infections are known to trigger Th1 responses, several studies have evaluated the efficacy of heat-killed Mycobacterium vaccae (HKMV) vaccination in the treatment of AD. In a randomized, double-blind, placebo-controlled trial involving children aged 5 to 18 years with moderate to severe AD, Arkwright and David[81] showed that a single-dose injection of HKMV (SRL172) significantly decreased involved areas and dermatitis score at a 3-month follow-up, whereas there was no significant change in the group

treated with placebo. In an attempt to replicate these results, 2 larger randomized, double-blind, placebo-controlled studies involving patients with AD of similar age range and disease severity using intradermal injection of HKMV or its derivative were performed. In one study, Berth-Jones and colleagues[82] found that a single intradermal injection of HKMV (SRP299) did not result in significant difference between the groups taking HKMV and placebo in affected surface areas, dermatitis score, or quality of life at a 3- or 6-month follow-up. More recently, Brothers and colleagues[83] used 3 intradermal injections of a derivative of HKMV (AVAC) at a biweekly interval. These investigators also found no significant difference between the groups in affected surface areas, dermatitis score, or quality of life at 3- and 6-month follow-up. In addition, in a younger age group (2–6 years) with moderate to severe AD, another double-blind, placebo-controlled study failed to confirm the efficacy of HKMV (SRP299).[84] Spontaneous improvement of AD was noted in both groups, consistent with the natural history of this disease.

Antipruritic Therapy

Opioid receptor antagonist

A double-blind, placebo-controlled trial of adult patients with AD using a topical naltrexone cream 1% showed that the cream had a significantly quicker onset of itch relief compared with placebo.[85] More recently, Malekzad and colleagues[86] showed that oral naltrexone significantly decreased itch, as measured by VAS, in a double-blind, placebo-controlled study of adult patients with AD. The subjects were given 25 mg of naltrexone or placebo capsules twice daily for 2 weeks, and VAS was measured at baseline, 1 week, and 2 weeks. There was no significant difference in VAS between the 2 groups at baseline, but the naltrexone group had significantly decreased VASs at 1 week and 2 weeks compared with the placebo ($P<.005$ and $P<.001$, respectively). Side effects in the group treated with naltrexone included dizziness, nausea, vomiting, headache, and cramps.

Selective serotonin reuptake inhibitors (SSRIs) have been proposed to have some effects on opioid receptors. In an open-label study involving 72 patients with pruritus of various conditions (of which only 3 subjects had AD), 2 SSRIs (paroxetine and fluvoxamine) had anti-itch effects in 68% of the patients.[87] Subjects with AD were among the subgroup of patients who had the best response. Further controlled studies specifically in patients with AD need to be conducted.

Anti–IL-31

IL-31 is produced primarily by Th2 cells and has been implicated in the pruritus associated with AD.[88] In a mouse model of AD, Grimstad and colleagues[89] showed that monoclonal anti–IL-31 antibody injection significantly decreased scratching behavior over a period of 7 weeks. The study illustrates the potential use of an IL-31 blocker as an antipruritic agent in AD, although studies need to be done in humans.

Semaphorin3A

In a study with skin biopsy specimens, Tominaga and colleagues[90] showed that there is decreased expression of semaphorin3A (Sema3A) and increased density of epidermal nerve fibers in the skin of patients with AD compared with that in healthy individuals. These investigators hypothesized that Sema3A may regulate the growth of nerve fibers that innervate the skin of patients with AD. In a murine model, Yamaguchi and colleagues[91] showed that injection of Sema3A significantly decreased the density of cutaneous nerve fibers, and led to decreased scratching behavior and improvement of eczematous changes. Recently, psoralen-UV-A (PUVA) therapy was shown to modulate Sema3A and nerve growth factor in patients with AD, decreasing epidermal expression of nerve growth factor and increasing epidermal expression of Sema3A.[92] PUVA therapy in these patients led to decreased epidermal nerve density and VAS score, and clinical improvement of AD. Reciprocal expression of nerve growth factor and Sema3A and their correlation with AD symptoms suggests a potential therapeutic approach in treating the pruritus of AD by regulating the levels of these proteins.

SUMMARY

AD remains an important disease, and it cannot be controlled in all patients with conventional therapies. The reasons for this are complex and include difficulty avoiding triggers, lack of understanding of skin care, suboptimal adherence with prescribed medications, limitations of medications due to adverse effects, and inadequate response to prescribed therapy. New insights into the complex pathogenesis of AD will likely lead to more targeted treatment for this disease. Novel therapies will likely emerge based on our increasing understanding of unique phenotypes of AD. Of note, filaggrin mutations have been shown to predispose to allergic inflammation in a mouse model.[93] Future antimicrobial approaches in AD may involve modulation of AMP expression. Specific therapies directed at pruritus in AD that lack the adverse effects of current therapies are needed because these symptoms continue to affect the quality of life of patients and their families.

REFERENCES

1. Odhiambo JA, Williams HC, Clayton TO, et al. Global variations in prevalence of eczema symptoms in children from ISAAC Phase Three. J Allergy Clin Immunol 2009;124:1251–8.
2. Faught J, Bierl C, Barton B, et al. Stress in mothers of young children with eczema. Arch Dis Child 2007;92:683–6.
3. Brenninkmeijer EE, Legierse CM, Sillevis Smitt JH, et al. The course of life of patients with childhood atopic dermatitis. Pediatr Dermatol 2009;26:14–22.
4. Boguniewicz M, Abramovits W, Paller A, et al. A multiple-domain framework of clinical, economic, and patient-reported outcomes for evaluating benefits of intervention in atopic dermatitis. J Drugs Dermatol 2007;6:416–23.
5. Ellis CN, Drake LA, Prendergast MM, et al. Cost of atopic dermatitis and eczema in the United States. J Am Acad Dermatol 2002;46:361–70.
6. Cork MJ, Danby SG, Vasilopoulos Y, et al. Epidermal barrier dysfunction in atopic dermatitis. J Invest Dermatol 2009;129:1892–908.
7. Leung DYM, Boguniewicz M, Howell M, et al. New insights into atopic dermatitis. J Clin Invest 2004;113:651–7.
8. Boguniewicz M, Leung DY. Recent insights into atopic dermatitis and implications for management of infectious complications. J Allergy Clin Immunol 2010;125: 4–13.
9. Ong P, Boguniewicz M. Atopic dermatitis. In: Katial R, editor. Primary care: clinics in office practice, 35. Philadelphia: Elsevier; 2008. p. 105–17.
10. Akdis CA, Akdis M, Bieber T, et al. Diagnosis and treatment of atopic dermatitis in children and adults: European Academy of Allergology and Clinical Immunology/ American Academy of Allergy, Asthma and Immunology/PRACTALL Consensus Report. J Allergy Clin Immunol 2006;118:152–69.
11. Charman CR, Morris AD, Williams HC. Topical corticosteroid phobia in patients with atopic eczema. Br J Dermatol 2000;142:931–6.

12. Krejci-Manwaring J, Tusa MG, Carroll C, et al. Stealth monitoring of adherence to topical medication: adherence is very poor in children with atopic dermatitis. J Am Acad Dermatol 2007;56:211–6.
13. Zuberbier Zuberbier T, Orlow SJ, Paller AS, et al. Patient perspectives on the management of atopic dermatitis. J Allergy Clin Immunol 2006;118:226–32.
14. Fonacier L, Spergel J, Charlesworth EN, et al. Report of the Topical Calcineurin Task Force of the American College of Allergy, Asthma and Immunology and the American Academy of Allergy, Asthma and Immunology. J Allergy Clin Immunol 2005;115:1249–53.
15. Arellano FM, Wentworth CE, Arana A, et al. Risk of lymphoma following exposure to calcineurin inhibitors and topical steroids in patients with atopic dermatitis. J Invest Dermatol 2007;127:808–16.
16. Orlow SJ. Topical calcineurin inhibitors in pediatric atopic dermatitis: a critical analysis of current issues. Paediatr Drugs 2007;9:289–99.
17. Ong PY. Emerging drugs for atopic dermatitis. Expert Opin Emerg Drugs 2009; 14:165–79.
18. Sugarman JL, Parish LC. Efficacy of a lipid-based barrier repair formulation in moderate-to-severe pediatric atopic dermatitis. J Drugs Dermatol 2009;8: 1106–11.
19. BuBmann C, Bieber T, Novak N. Systemic therapeutic options for severe atopic dermatitis. J Dtsch Dermatol Ges 2009;7:205–19.
20. Gambichler T. Management of atopic dermatitis using photo(chemo)therapy. Arch Dermatol Res 2009;301:197–203.
21. Devillers AC, Oranje AP. Efficacy and safety of 'wet-wrap' dressings as an intervention treatment in children with severe and/or refractory atopic dermatitis: a critical review of the literature. Br J Dermatol 2006;154:579–85.
22. Boguniewicz M, Nicol NH, Kelsay K, et al. A multidisciplinary approach to evaluation and treatment of atopic dermatitis. Semin Cutan Med Surg 2008;27:117–27.
23. Loden M, Andersson AC, Lindberg M. Improvement in skin barrier function in patients with atopic dermatitis after treatment with a moisturizing cream (Canoderm). Br J Dermatol 1999;140:264–7.
24. Kezic S, Kemperman PM, Koster ES, et al. Loss-of-function mutations in the filaggrin gene lead to reduced level of natural moisturizing factor in the stratum corneum. J Invest Dermatol 2008;128:2117–9.
25. Wirén K, Nohlgård C, Nyberg F, et al. Treatment with a barrier-strengthening moisturizing cream delays relapse of atopic dermatitis: a prospective and randomized controlled clinical trial. J Eur Acad Dermatol Venereol 2009;23:1267–72.
26. Grether-Beck S, Mühlberg K, Brenden H, et al. Bioactive molecules from the Blue Lagoon: in vitro and in vivo assessment of silica mud and microalgae extracts for their effects on skin barrier function and prevention of skin ageing. Exp Dermatol 2008;17:771–9.
27. Schlievert PM, Strandberg KL, Lin YC, et al. Secreted virulence factor comparison between methicillin-resistant and methicillin-sensitive *Staphylococcus aureus* and its relevance to atopic dermatitis. J Allergy Clin Immunol 2010;125: 39–49.
28. Fluhr JW, Breternitz M, Kowatzki D, et al. Silver-loaded seaweed-based cellulosic fiber improves epidermal skin physiology in atopic dermatitis: safety assessment, mode of action and controlled, randomized single-blinded exploratory in vivo study. Exp Dermatol 2009. [Epub ahead of print].
29. Lai Y, Di Nardo A, Nakatsuji T, et al. Commensal bacteria regulate Toll-like receptor 3-dependent inflammation after skin injury. Nat Med 2009;15:1377–82.

30. Huang JT, Abrams M, Tlougan B, et al. Treatment of *Staphylococcus aureus* colonization in atopic dermatitis decreases disease severity. Pediatrics 2009; 123:e808–14.
31. Wohlrab J, Jost G, Abeck D. Antiseptic efficacy of a low-dosed topical triclosan/ chlorhexidine combination therapy in atopic dermatitis. Skin Pharmacol Physiol 2007;20:71–6.
32. Tan WP, Suresh S, Tey HL, et al. A randomized double-blind controlled trial to compare a triclosan-containing emollient with vehicle for the treatment of atopic dermatitis. Clin Exp Dermatol 2010;35:e109–12.
33. Wang R, Braughton KR, Kretschmer D, et al. Identification of novel cytolytic peptides as key virulence determinants for community-associated MRSA. Nat Med 2007;13:1510–4.
34. Park J, Jagasia R, Kaufmann GF, et al. Infection control by antibody disruption of bacterial quorum sensing signaling. Chem Biol 2007;14:1119–27.
35. Otto M. Targeted immunotherapy for staphylococcal infections: focus on anti-MSCRAMM antibodies. BioDrugs 2008;22:27–36.
36. Stranger-Jones YK, Bae T, Schneewind O. Vaccine assembly from surface proteins of *Staphylococcus aureus*. Proc Natl Acad Sci U S A 2006;103:16942–7.
37. Clarke SR, Brummell KJ, Horsburgh MJ, et al. Identification of in vivo-expressed antigens of *Staphylococcus aureus* and their use in vaccinations for protection against nasal carriage. J Infect Dis 2006;193:1098–108.
38. Weidenmaier C, Kokai-Kun JF, Kristian SA, et al. Role of teichoic acids in *Staphylococcus aureus* nasal colonization, a major risk factor in nosocomial infections. Nat Med 2004;10:243–5.
39. Travers JB, Kozman A, Mousdicas N, et al. Infected atopic dermatitis lesions contain pharmacologic amounts of lipoteichoic acid. J Allergy Clin Immunol 2010;125:146–52.e1–2.
40. Buonpane RA, Churchill HR, Moza B, et al. Neutralization of staphylococcal enterotoxin B by soluble, high-affinity receptor antagonists. Nat Med 2007;13: 725–9.
41. Yang X, Buonpane RA, Moza B, et al. Neutralization of multiple staphylococcal superantigens by a single-chain protein consisting of affinity-matured, variable domain repeats. J Invest Dermatol 2008;198:344–8.
42. Vora S, Damon I, Fulginiti V, et al. Severe eczema vaccinatum in a household contact of a smallpox vaccinee. Clin Infect Dis 2008;46:1555–61.
43. Howell MD, Gallo RL, Boguniewicz M, et al. Cytokine milieu of atopic dermatitis skin subverts the innate immune response to vaccinia virus. Immunity 2006;24: 341–8.
44. Howell MD, Streib JE, Leung DY. Antiviral activity of human beta-defensin 3 against vaccinia virus. J Allergy Clin Immunol 2007;119:1022–5.
45. Savage PB, Li C, Taotafa U, et al. Antibacterial properties of cationic steroid antibiotics. FEMS Microbiol Lett 2002;217:1–7.
46. Ding B, Taotofa U, Orsak T, et al. Synthesis and characterization of peptide-cationic steroid antibiotic conjugates. Org Lett 2004;6:3433–6.
47. Howell MD, Streib JE, Kim BE, et al. Ceragenins: a class of antiviral compounds to treat orthopox infections. J Invest Dermatol 2009;129:2668–75.
48. Lonsdorf AS, Hwang ST, Enk AH. Chemokine receptors in T-cell-mediated diseases of the skin. J Invest Dermatol 2009;129:2552–66.
49. Ong PY, Ferdman RM, Dunaway T, et al. Down-regulation of atopic dermatitis-associated serum chemokines by wet-wrap treatment: a pilot study. Ann Allergy Asthma Immunol 2008;100:286–7.

50. Nakagami Y, Kawashima K, Yonekubo K, et al. Novel CC chemokine receptor 4 antagonist RS-1154 inhibits ovalbumin-induced ear swelling in mice. Eur J Pharmacol 2009;624:38–44.

51. Willems LI, Ijzerman AP. Small molecule antagonists for chemokine CCR3 receptors. Med Res Rev 2009. [Epub ahead of print].

52. Suzuki K, Morokata T, Morihira K, et al. In vitro and in vivo characterization of a novel CCR3 antagonist, YM-344031. Biochem Biophys Res Commun 2006; 339:1217–23.

53. Igawa K, Satoh T, Yokozeki H. A therapeutic effect of STAT6 decoy oligodeoxynucleotide ointment in atopic dermatitis: a pilot study in adults. Br J Dermatol 2009; 160:1124–6.

54. Groves RW, Wilbraham D, Fuller R, et al. Inhibition of IL-4 and IL-13 with an IL-4 mutein (Aeroderm) protects against flares in atopic eczema. J Invest Dermatol 2007;127:S54.

55. Morioka T, Yamanaka K, Mori H, et al. IL-4/IL-13 antagonist DNA vaccination successfully suppresses Th2 type chronic dermatitis. Br J Dermatol 2009;160: 1172–9.

56. Kimata H. Selective enhancement of production of IgE, IgG4, and Th2-cell cytokine during the rebound phenomenon in atopic dermatitis and prevention by suplatast tosilate. Ann Allergy Asthma Immunol 1999;82:293–5.

57. Murakami T, Yamanaka K, Tokime K, et al. Topical suplatast tosilate (IPD) ameliorates Th2 cytokine-mediated dermatitis in caspase-1 transgenic mice by downregulating interleukin-4 and interleukin-5. Br J Dermatol 2006;155: 27–32.

58. Miyachi Y, Katayama I, Furue M. Suplatast/tacrolimus combination therapy for refractory facial erythema in adult patients with atopic dermatitis: a meta-analysis study. Allergol Int 2007;56:269–75.

59. Behshad R, Cooper KD, Korman NJ. A retrospective case series review of the peroxisome proliferator-activated receptor ligand rosiglitazone in the treatment of atopic dermatitis. Arch Dermatol 2008;144:84–8.

60. Staumont-Sallé D, Abboud G, Brénuchon C, et al. Peroxisome proliferator-activated receptor alpha regulates skin inflammation and humoral response in atopic dermatitis. J Allergy Clin Immunol 2008;121:962–8.

61. Hatano Y, Man MQ, Uchida Y, et al. Murine atopic dermatitis responds to peroxisome proliferator-activated receptors alpha and beta/delta (but not gamma) and liver X receptor activators. J Allergy Clin Immunol 2010;125: 160–9.e1–5.

62. De Vry CG, Valdez M, Lazarov M, et al. Topical application of a novel immunomodulatory peptide, RDP58, reduces skin inflammation in the phorbol ester-induced dermatitis model. J Invest Dermatol 2005;125:473–81.

63. Takei S, Arora YK, Walker SM. Intravenous immunoglobulin contains specific antibodies inhibitory to activation of T cells by staphylococcal toxin superantigens. J Clin Invest 1993;91:602–7.

64. Jolles S. A review of high-dose intravenous immunoglobulin treatment for atopic dermatitis. Clin Exp Dermatol 2002;27:3–7.

65. Holgate S, Casale T, Wenzel S, et al. The anti-inflammatory effects of omalizumab confirm the central role of IgE in allergic inflammation. J Allergy Clin Immunol 2005;115:459–65.

66. Vigo PG, Girgis KR, Pfuetze BL, et al. Efficacy of anti-IgE therapy in patients with atopic dermatitis therapy on cutaneous symptoms of AD. J Am Acad Dermatol 2006;55:168–70.

67. Krathen RA, Hsu S. Failure of omalizumab for treatment of severe adult atopic dermatitis. J Am Acad Dermatol 2005;53:338–40.
68. Lane JE, Cheyney JM, Lane TN, et al. Treatment of recalcitrant atopic dermatitis with omalizumab. J Am Acad Dermatol 2006;54:68–72.
69. Belloni B, Ziai M, Lim A, et al. Low-dose anti-IgE therapy in patients with atopic eczema with high serum IgE levels. J Allergy Clin Immunol 2007;120:1223–5.
70. Werfel T, Breuer K, Rueff F, et al. Usefulness of specific immunotherapy in patients with atopic dermatitis and allergic sensitization to house dust mites: a multi-centre, randomized, dose-response study. Allergy 2006;61:202–5.
71. Bussmann C, Maintz L, Hart J, et al. Clinical improvement and immunological changes in atopic dermatitis patients undergoing subcutaneous immuno-therapy with a house dust mite allergoid: a pilot study. Clin Exp Allergy 2007;37:1277–85.
72. Pajno GB, Caminiti L, Vita D, et al. Sublingual immunotherapy in mite-sensitized children with atopic dermatitis: a randomized, double-blind, placebo-controlled study. J Allergy Clin Immunol 2007;120:164–70.
73. Katayama I, Minatohara K, Yokozeki H, et al. Topical vitamin D3 downregulates IgE-mediated murine biphasic cutaneous reactions. Int Arch Allergy Immunol 1996;111(1):71–6.
74. Li M, Hener P, Zhang Z, et al. Topical vitamin D3 and low-calcemic analogs induce thymic stromal lymphopoietin in mouse keratinocytes and trigger an atopic dermatitis. Proc Natl Acad Sci U S A 2006;103:11736–41.
75. Vähävihu K, Ylianttila L, Salmelin R, et al. Heliotherapy improves vitamin D balance and atopic dermatitis. Br J Dermatol 2008;158:1323–8.
76. Autio P, Komulainen P, Larni HM. Heliotherapy in atopic dermatitis: a prospective study on climatotherapy using the SCORAD index. Acta Derm Venereol 2002;82:436–40.
77. Sidbury R, Sullivan AF, Thadhani RI, et al. Randomized controlled trial of vitamin D supplementation for winter-related atopic dermatitis in Boston: a pilot study. Br J Dermatol 2008;159:245–7.
78. Ong PY, Ohtake T, Brandt C, et al. Endogenous antimicrobial peptides and skin infections in atopic dermatitis. N Engl J Med 2002;347:1151–60.
79. Christophers E, Henseler T. Contrasting disease patterns in psoriasis and atopic dermatitis. Arch Dermatol Res 1987;279:S48–51.
80. Hata TR, Kotol P, Jackson M, et al. Administration of oral vitamin D induces cath-elicidin production in atopic individuals. J Allergy Clin Immunol 2008;122:829–31.
81. Arkwright PD, David TJ. Intradermal administration of a killed *Mycobacterium vaccae* suspension (SRL 172) is associated with improvement in atopic derma-titis in children with moderate-to-severe disease. J Allergy Clin Immunol 2001;107:531–4.
82. Berth-Jones J, Arkwright PD, Marasovic D, et al. Killed *Mycobacterium vaccae* suspension in children with moderate-to-severe atopic dermatitis: a randomized, double-blind, placebo-controlled trial. Clin Exp Allergy 2006;36:1115–21.
83. Brothers S, Asher MI, Jaksic M, et al. Effect of a *Mycobacterium vaccae* deriva-tive on paediatric atopic dermatitis: a randomized, controlled trial. Clin Exp Der-matol 2009;34:770–5.
84. Arkwright PD, David TJ. Effect of *Mycobacterium vaccae* on atopic dermatitis in children of different ages. Br J Dermatol 2003;149:1029–34.
85. Bigliardi PL, Stammer H, Jost G, et al. Treatment of pruritus with topically applied opiate receptor antagonist. J Am Acad Dermatol 2007;56:979–88.

86. Malekzad F, Arbabi M, Mohtasham N, et al. Efficacy of oral naltrexone on pruritus in atopic eczema: a double-blind, placebo-controlled study. J Eur Acad Dermatol Venereol 2009;23:948–50.
87. Ständer S, Böckenholt B, Schürmeyer-Horst F, et al. Treatment of chronic pruritus with the selective serotonin re-uptake inhibitors paroxetine and fluvoxamine: results of an open-labelled, two-arm proof-of-concept study. Acta Derm Venereol 2009;89:45–51.
88. Sonkoly E, Muller A, Lauerma AI, et al. IL-31: a new link between T cells and pruritus in atopic skin inflammation. J Allergy Clin Immunol 2006;117:411–7.
89. Grimstad O, Sawanobori Y, Vestergaard C, et al. Anti-interleukin-31-antibodies ameliorate scratching behaviour in NC/Nga mice: a model of atopic dermatitis. Exp Dermatol 2009;18:35–43.
90. Tominaga M, Ogawa H, Takamori K. Decreased production of semaphorin 3A in the lesional skin of atopic dermatitis. Br J Dermatol 2008;158:842–4.
91. Yamaguchi J, Nakamura F, Aihara M, et al. Semaphorin3A alleviates skin lesions and scratching behavior in NC/Nga mice, an atopic dermatitis model. J Invest Dermatol 2008;128:2842–9.
92. Tominaga M, Tengara S, Kamo A, et al. Psoralen-ultraviolet A therapy alters epidermal Sema3A and NGF levels and modulates epidermal innervation in atopic dermatitis. J Dermatol Sci 2009;55:40–6.
93. Fallon PG, Sasaki T, Sandilands A, et al. A homozygous frameshift mutation in the mouse Flg gene facilitates enhanced percutaneous allergen priming. Nat Genet 2009;41:602–8.

Index

Note: Page numbers of article titles are in **boldface** type.

Immunol Allergy Clin N Am 30 (2010) 441–451
doi:10.1016/S0889-8561(10)00061-5
0889-8561/10/$ – see front matter © 2010 Elsevier Inc. All rights reserved.

immunology.theclinics.com

Printed and bound by CPI Group (UK) Ltd, Croydon, CR0 4YY

03/10/2024

01040456-0016